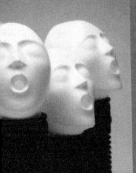

Canadian
First Aid Manual

With the 2015
CPR guidelines

LIFESAVING SOCIETY

The Lifeguarding Experts

THE 2015 RESUSCITATION GUIDELINES

Every five years, based on a review of the best evidence available, the International Liaison Committee on Resuscitation (ILCOR) and the American Heart Association (AHA) announce changes to the Guidelines for CPR & Emergency Cardiovascular Care (ECC). The changes are designed to make it easier for rescuers and health care providers alike to learn, remember and perform better CPR.

The most recent changes were announced in October 2015. They continue to emphasize that better outcomes and survival rates result from quick recognition, rapid activation of the emergency medical system and the application of effective CPR. This means:

- *Push hard, push fast:* forceful, fast compressions provide better circulation of blood and oxygen. This means 100–120 compressions/minute and, for adults, a depth of 5–6 cm/2–2.4 inches.
- *Minimize interruption in chest compressions:* blood flow stops if compressions stop.
- *Early defibrillation:* victims have a better chance of surviving when CPR is performed in combination with early defibrillation.

The 2015 guidelines continue to emphasize starting CPR with compressions rather than rescue breaths for cardiac arrest victims. With drowning victims however, rescuers continue to start CPR with breaths because drowning victims need oxygen as soon as possible.

ACKNOWLEDGEMENTS

Many knowledgeable and generous individuals participated in the development of the *Canadian First Aid Manual.* In particular we wish to thank: Brook Beatty, Rebecca Boyd, Brian Cartwright, Anne McMillan, J.P. Molin, Peter Mumford, Larry Patterson, Paula Stevens and Wilkie Soo.

The Society's medical advisors also made valuable contributions in the development of the text: Dr. Steve Beerman, MD, CCFP, FCFP, chair of the Medical Committee of the International Life Saving Federation; Alberta & NWT Medical Advisor Dr. William Patton, MD, CCFP (EM), and Ontario Medical Advisory Chair Carl Rotmann.

We thank our photographer Adrian Herscovici and models: Brook Beatty, Andrea Chow, Jeremey Ludwig, Melissa Spano, Shawn Wannop, Yung Yung Wong, Roman Zemtsov and Eric Zimmerman.

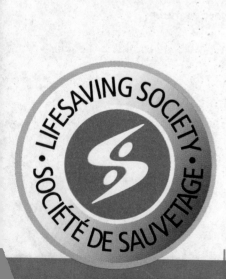

INTRODUCTION

Welcome to the Lifesaving Society's first aid training course and the *Canadian First Aid Manual*. Your interest in helping others is a worthy Canadian value, and the first aid skills you acquire will allow you to assist your family and community.

First aid training also increases your own personal safety. The knowledge you gain encourages healthy lifestyles as well as the prevention of accidents, injury and illness. Such prevention, and early effective treatment of injury and illness, may help reduce the expanding demands on our health care system.

First aid knowledge and skills are based on principles that can be adapted to many situations. The most important first aid skills are easy to learn and to apply: these include airway, breathing and circulation (ABCs) management, application of pressure for bleeding, stabilization of fractures, and recognition of shock. Practice of these basic skills is more important than the management of uncommon, less urgent scenarios.

Sophisticated emergency resources may be available in your community, but they will rarely be the first responder to victims of injury or illness. Experience tells us that if you are called upon to perform first aid in an emergency, it will likely be for someone you know or care about – a family member, friend or colleague – at home or in the workplace. When Emergency Medical Service *is* available, calling for assistance and providing reassurance may be the only service required for the victim.

Building the confidence to step forward in a stressful situation is a major objective in first aid training. While there may be many years between learning and application, the techniques you learn now are the skills you will apply when the need arises.

Practice and repetition of basic lifesaving information and skills maintains your confidence. Be sure to keep your skills up to date with practice, review and refresher courses.

Congratulations on choosing the Lifesaving Society first aid program. We are confident the skills you learn will make a difference.

Steve Beerman, M.D., CCFP, FCFP
past President, International Life Saving Federation;
past Chair, ILS Medical Commission;
past President, Lifesaving Society Canada

CONTENTS

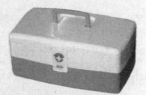

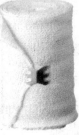

Secondary Emergencies

AED and Airway Management

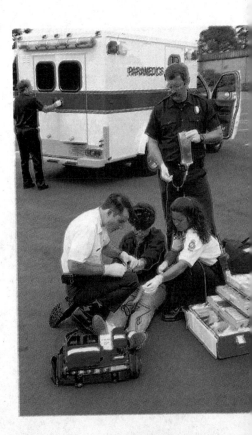

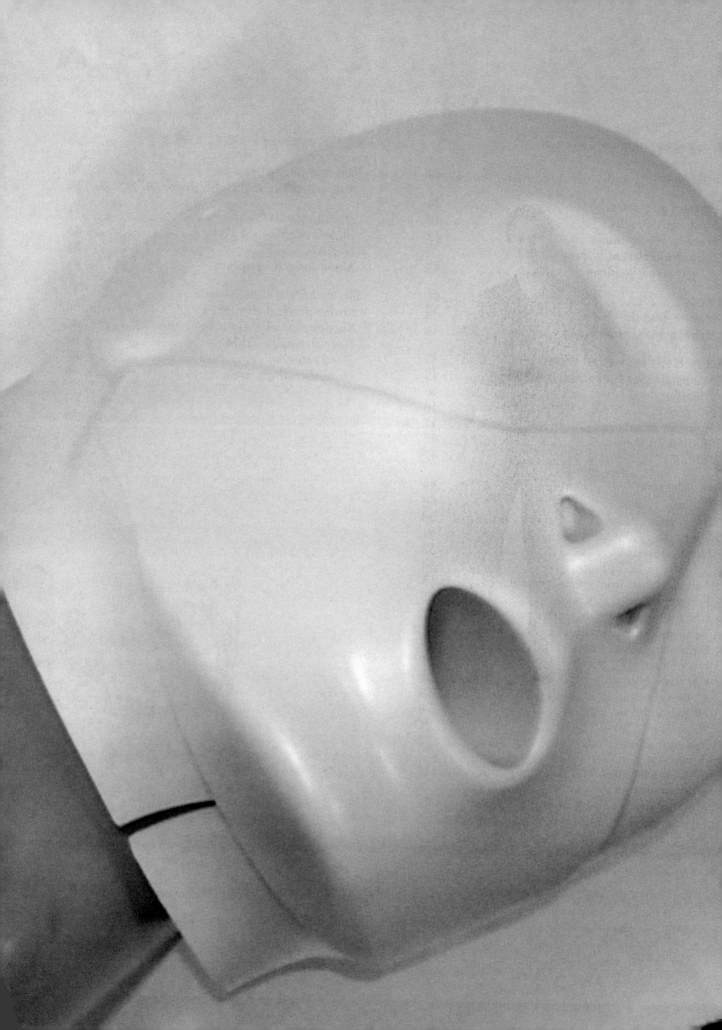

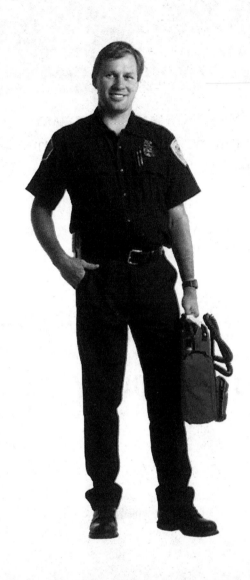

Introduction to First Aid

PREVENTION

The simplest prevention strategy is to avoid doing things that cause mishaps and injury. But this strategy isn't always practical. What is practical is to learn about the risks involved in activities in which you participate and manage those risks to prevent injury.

Many serious injuries resulting from accidents are preventable. Researchers can identify patterns of behaviour and common causes for particular injuries by analyzing the circumstances that lead to injuries. An accident can then be traced back to its cause, making it quite predictable and not necessarily "accidental."

GOALS OF FIRST AID

FIRST AID IS THE IMMEDIATE AND TEMPORARY CARE OF ILLNESS OR INJURY. THE GOALS OF FIRST AID ARE EXPRESSED IN THE "3 Ps":

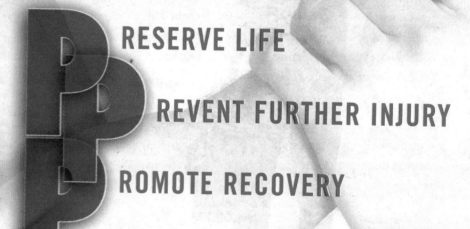

PRESERVE LIFE

PREVENT FURTHER INJURY

PROMOTE RECOVERY

FIRST AIDERS IN THE COMMUNITY

Who is a first aider?

A first aider is someone at an emergency scene who suspects injury or illness and provides first aid to preserve life, prevent further injury and promote recovery. As a first aider, you take charge of emergency scenes; calm and reassure people, protect victims and their belongings, and take steps to help victims get medical attention.

First aiders do not *diagnose*, nor do they provide medical help – medical help is given by a medical doctor, nurse or paramedic.

First aiders and the Emergency Medical System (EMS)

The Emergency Medical System (EMS) is a community-wide system for responding to emergencies. It consists of police, fire and ambulance services. Your role as a first aider in an emergency that requires medical help is to:

- activate the system with a telephone call
- care for the victim while waiting

(Read details about contacting EMS under *Recruiting Assistance*.)

First aiders and the workplace

Many employers identify or designate workers with first aid training. Some companies also assess general first aid practices and formalize them into company procedures that fit the nature of the work and worksite. Such procedures must meet or exceed local regulations for health and safety.

If you become a designated first aider, ask for a complete orientation to learn what is required by law and by the company.

1) Gain permission if the victim is conscious.

2) Act reasonably within the scope of your training.

3) Continue until someone more qualified takes over unless you are at risk or exhausted.

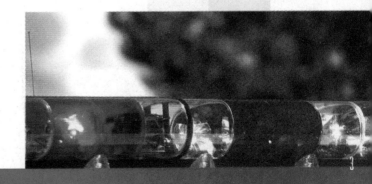

DO NOT RESUSCITATE (DNR) ORDERS

A DNR order is a written formal statement communicating a person's decision to decline resuscitation should they stop breathing. These orders may appear within other documents such as "advanced directives" or "living wills."

DNR orders* are rare in first aid situations. First aiders should proceed with CPR if required unless presented with a DNR order.

If first aid is part of your duties as an employee (e.g. lifeguards), ask your employer if they have specific guidelines or policies related to DNR orders and follow them.

---

* Ontario's Workplace Safety & Insurance Board advises that DNR orders are not valid for first aiders in Ontario.

First aiders and the law

Legislation: Most provinces have an act such as Alberta's Emergency Medical Aid Act or Ontario's Good Samaritan Act. These protect first aiders from liability for damages allegedly caused by their first aid assistance (through a careless act or omission). These laws cover situations where the first aider acts voluntarily outside the scope of employment, is at the scene of the incident, and is providing first aid to the best of their trained ability.

Standard of care: If there are any questions about the level (or standard) of care you provided, the court asks the general question, "What would a reasonable person with your training do under the same circumstances?" As long as you do what you were trained to do, you are protected by the law.

When to start: If the victim is conscious, identify yourself as a first aider and ask permission to help. Say something like, "I know first aid, may I help you?" This builds trust and rapport.

Minors require a different approach. Seek permission from the child's parent or guardian if they are present.

When to stop: Once you begin first aid, the law expects you to continue until:
a) another qualified person takes over
b) you become too exhausted to continue
c) you are at personal risk
d) EMS or other medical personnel (e.g. a doctor) assume responsibility

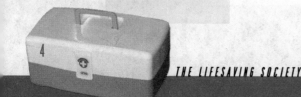

FIRST AID AND RESCUE PROCESS

THE PROCESS OF HELPING PEOPLE IN TROUBLE IS DYNAMIC, IN THE SENSE THAT YOU REPEAT THE RESCUE ELEMENTS – RECOGNIZE, ASSESS, ACT – DURING EACH PHASE OF THE RESCUE. A RESCUER APPLIES EACH OF THESE RESCUE ELEMENTS IN EACH OF THE RESCUE PHASES:

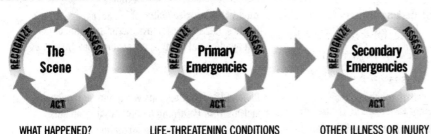

WHAT HAPPENED?   LIFE-THREATENING CONDITIONS   OTHER ILLNESS OR INJURY

Rescue phases

Respond to any rescue situation in the following order:

1. **The Scene** – deal with immediate environmental threats.

2. **Primary Emergencies** – handle life-threatening emergency priorities of breathing and circulation.

3. **Secondary Emergencies** – care for other injuries and illness.

Continue to provide ongoing victim care until hand over.

Rescue elements

These three elements ensure the care of the victim is appropriate to the situation:

1. **Recognize:** Recognition is the ability to identify when someone is hurt, sick, or in a dangerous situation. It involves observing the circumstances of the emergency and monitoring the situation.

2. **Assess:** Assessment is a deliberate search for clues to help you decide what to do. It is pivotal to first aid and will guide your actions in an emergency. Assessment can take a number of forms – a look around, a question or series of questions, checking vital signs, evaluating signs and symptoms, and completing a head-to-toe examination. It can be directed to the environment, witnesses and victim.

3. **Act:** Action is determined by the assessment. The act of treating injuries is one response to the assessment, but action also refers to doing things like removing hazards, directing bystanders and calling for help. In some cases "no action" is appropriate. Because each emergency presents a unique set of conditions, the sequence of actions is different in every situation.

Combining the phases and elements

Altogether, follow these steps:

- **Scene** – recognize, assess, act on the assessment.

- **Primary emergencies** – recognize, assess, act on the assessment.

- **Secondary emergencies** – recognize, assess, act on the assessment.

A first aider's role does not end after first aid is administered. Unless you are in danger, or physically unable, it is necessary to control the emergency scene until someone more qualified takes over. Keep the victim(s) in the best possible condition and provide ongoing care. This includes things such as treating for shock, offering reassurance, loosening tight clothing and monitoring vital signs.

STEP-BY-STEP

always follow these steps. Insert specific techniques and procedures as described in later sections.

Recognize ⫸	Assess ⫸	Act
THE SCENE		
When someone is injured, ill or in danger... then proceed.	**Hazards check** Is it safe? **Mechanism of injury** What happened? Is there a head/spinal injury?	☐ Shout for help; attract attention. ☐ Introduce yourself as a first aider. ☐ Gain permission to help. ☐ Remove hazards or remove victim from hazards. ☐ If a head/spinal injury is suspected, then treat it as such.
PRIMARY EMERGENCIES (Recognize – Assess – Act)		
When both you and the victim are safe from environmental hazards... then proceed.	**LOC** Level of consciousness **ABC** **Airway, Breathing, Circulation** (quick, visual check for absent or abnormal [e.g., gasping] breathing, coughing, movement, bleeding or shock).	☐ Phone EMS for unresponsive victims or responsive victims with breathing or circulation problems. ☐ Treat ABC emergencies immediately. ☐ Treat for shock.
SECONDARY EMERGENCIES Complete assessment to end of the head-to-toe exam, then act		
When the victim is breathing and ABC emergencies treated... then proceed.	**Victim history** **Incident history** Talk to victim, witnesses and look around. **Vital signs (Vitals)** LOC, breathing, circulation, skin, pupils. **Head-to-toe examination** Medical condition identification. Distal circulation. Distal sensation. Head-to-toe exam. **Vitals check every 5–10 min.** Monitor for change.	☐ Record relevant information. ☐ History ☐ Vital signs ☐ Injuries ☐ Treat conditions, starting with the most serious. ☐ Continue treating for shock. ☐ Be prepared to respond to any changes.

Ongoing victim care throughout the process:

Communicate
- ☐ Reassure victim.
- ☐ Ask questions.
- ☐ Describe what you are doing.

Prevent disease transmission
- ☐ Wear gloves, use barrier devices.
- ☐ Wash hands and clean up appropriately.

Recruit bystanders

Treatment – treat for cause of shock, illness or injury – (WARTS)
- ☐ **W**armth.
- ☐ **A**BCs – loosen clothing, monitor vital signs.
- ☐ **R**est and Reassurance.
- ☐ **T**reatment – treat for cause of shock.
- ☐ **S**emi-prone (recovery) position.

At the end:

Stop treatment when
- ☐ EMS personnel assume responsibility or another qualified person takes over.
- ☐ You are at personal risk or are physically unable to continue.

Worksite injury?
- ☐ Complete incident report form if required.

Critical Incident Stress
- ☐ Recognize your feelings and responses.
- ☐ Talk about the emergency event.

THE LIFESAVING SOCIETY

RECRUITING ASSISTANCE

When to get medical assistance

PHONING FOR MEDICAL CARE MAY BE THE GREATEST LIFESAVING MEASURE YOU TAKE. BUT WHO SHOULD YOU CALL AND WHEN? THIS CHART LISTS THE GENERAL RULES.

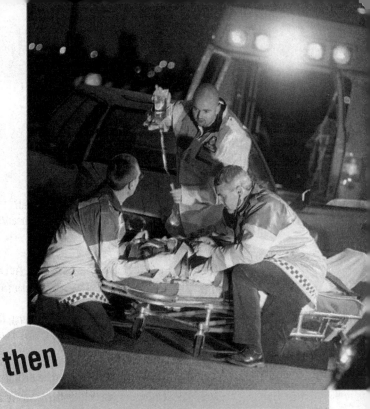

if

then

The victim is unresponsive either at the beginning or in the middle of providing care.

Phone EMS immediately

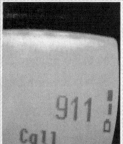

The victim shows signs of:
- breathing or circulation problems
- a heart attack or stroke
- a spinal injury
- severe shock
- deteriorating vital signs
- a major injury
- confusion, disorientation

Phone EMS
Transport the victim to hospital by ambulance.

The victim needs medical attention for head injuries, bleeding, wounds, broken bones, asthma, seizures, heat exhaustion and other secondary emergencies.

Transport to hospital
- Phone EMS unless you have no other option.
- For children, give the parents the option.
- If a child's parents aren't immediately available, call EMS.

The incident has been treated as much as possible for the time being, but should really be checked further (e.g. minor burns, fainting, strains).

See a doctor
- If in doubt, phone EMS.
- Recommend that the victim seek medical attention and continue to monitor the situation.
- For children, advise the parents of the situation.

The incident is minor and has been treated adequately for today. It may require medical attention if it does not get better (e.g. insect stings, sunburn, small wounds, pressure squeeze).

Monitor the situation
- Recommend that the victim monitor the situation and if it gets worse, seek medical attention.

EMS

The Emergency Medical System* (EMS) is a community-wide system for responding to emergencies. It consists of police, fire and ambulance services. Knowing the EMS telephone number for your community or worksite will save you time in an emergency.

Contacting EMS (finding the right phone number): Many communities use 911, but some still have a separate telephone number for each emergency response service. If you don't know the number, dial "0" and ask the operator for help, or check the front pages of the telephone book.

Who should call: If possible, do not leave the victim alone. Send someone else to call EMS while you continue the first aid process. Give the caller the information listed below and tell the person to report back to you to confirm the call has been made.

The call – provide this information:
- the number of victims
- victim age, gender, condition
- the location where EMS should go

Stay on the line: Ask when EMS will arrive. Do not hang up until the EMS dispatcher tells you. This will ensure the call is not cut off before EMS has all the information needed to respond. Use speaker mode on your mobile device to follow instructions from the EMS dispatcher.

Meeting EMS on scene: After the EMS call is made, give someone the job of meeting the emergency team and directing them to the victim.

When EMS arrives: They assume responsibility for the care of the victim. EMS follow their own action plans and will ask for information as they need it. Stand by to respond to their questions as they work and provide assistance if necessary.

* EMS is also defined as Emergency Medical Services.

Bystanders

There is no need to act alone if bystanders are present. A firm, simple request for assistance will get you extra help. Bystanders can:
- phone EMS
- meet the EMS team and direct them to the scene
- help to immobilize the neck and head if a spinal injury is suspected
- remove hazards or help you move the victim to safety
- get blankets, first aid supplies or other equipment
- calm or comfort the victim
- protect the victim's personal belongings
- write down the vital signs, details of the incident and victim history
- ask any crowds that gather to stay back to leave space to work
- be taught what to do, to free you to move to another step

Some bystanders may have training or experience and can:
- perform rescue breathing or CPR
- provide first aid treatment
- check vital signs

Activating bystanders: Although people are usually willing to help, they can be hesitant about being the first one involved. Or they may think that everything is under control and they have nothing to offer. When speaking with bystanders, be assertive and direct so they understand your request. Here are some tips:
- ask for help
- identify the bystander(s) to whom you are speaking
- find out if bystanders have any lifesaving or first aid training
- give clear, specific instructions
- ask them to report to you when they have finished their task
- thank them when it is over

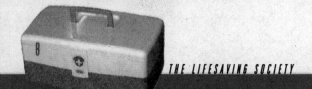

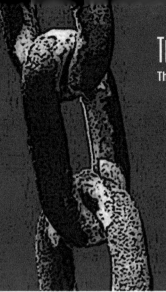

The Canadian Chain of Survival

The Canadian Chain of Survival links first aiders and EMS into a sequence of interventions intended to prevent, treat and support recovery of people who have suffered a stroke or heart disease.

Early recognition and EMS activation	Immediate recognition of cardiac arrest and activation of emergency response system.
Early CPR	Start CPR immediately if the victim is not breathing.
Early Defibrillation	To correct the beat if the heart is fibrillating.
Early Advanced Care	Access to medications and other medical treatments that can improve survival and quality of life.
Early Rehabilitation	To assist in the return to active life after a heart attack or stroke.

VICTIM CARRIES AND ASSISTS

IF YOU MUST MOVE A VICTIM, SELECT A METHOD THAT POSES THE LEAST RISK TO BOTH OF YOU. HERE ARE SOME LIFTING AND TRANSPORTATION TECHNIQUES TO USE WHEN MOVING A VICTIM AWAY FROM DANGER OR TOWARDS FURTHER TREATMENT AND COMFORT.

Walking assist – when the victim can walk but needs assistance over a short distance.

> **Starting position:** Both the rescuer and victim are standing facing the same direction.
> - Support the victim by placing one arm around his or her waist, and by putting the victim's arm closest to you over your shoulder. Walk at a pace that is comfortable for the victim.

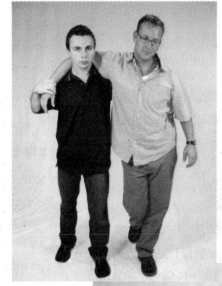

One-rescuer drag – when you are alone with an unconscious victim and you need to move a short distance quickly.

> **Starting position:** The victim is lying on his or her back.
> - Stand behind the victim's head, crouch to reach under his or her armpits, grab the wrists and pull them towards you so the arms cross.
> - Lift the victim up so that the heels drag. Pull and walk backwards.

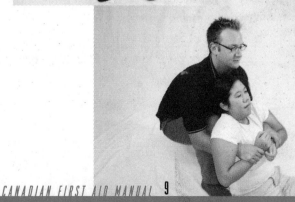

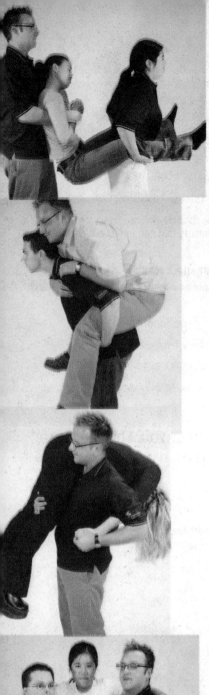

Two-rescuer carry – with an unconscious victim.

Starting position: The victim is lying on his or her back.

- First rescuer supports the upper body as in the one-rescuer drag.
- Second rescuer stands between the victim's legs and lifts, supporting the legs at the thigh. It is easiest to face the direction of travel.
- Travel in either direction, towards the head or the feet.

Pick-a-back carry – for a conscious victim who cannot walk, but needs to move quickly. Do NOT use this carry for victims with fractures or dislocations.

Starting position: The victim is standing or sitting.

- Squat in front of the victim with your back towards them.
- Ask the victim to hold on to your shoulders, and then to wrap his or her legs around your waist.
- Support the victim's legs under the thighs with your arms.
- Stand up and carry.

Over-one-shoulder carry (firefighter's carry) – when you are much larger than the victim or if you have ample strength.

Starting position: The victim is sitting or lying face up.

- Roll the victim over your shoulder. On your shoulder, the victim should be bent at the waist, legs in front of you.
- Hold on to the victim's legs, and hold on to one wrist over your other shoulder.
- Move slowly and deliberately – walking quickly may cause the victim to vomit.

Human chair (seat assists) – for two rescuers to transport a conscious person.

Starting position: The victim is lying down or sitting.

Two-hand seat:

- Rescuers crouch on either side of the victim and grab each other's wrists to create a seat for the victim to sit on.
- One set of locked wrists is behind the victim creating a backrest.
- The other set of locked wrists is under the victim's thighs creating a seat.
- Ask the victim to provide additional stability by reaching across and holding on to both rescuers' shoulders.

Four-hand seat:

- If the rescuers do not have enough grip strength for a lift with only two hands forming the seat, they can increase their strength by interlocking their four wrists to create a square seat.
- As above, the victim should hold on to the rescuers' shoulders for additional support and stability.

FIRST AID KITS

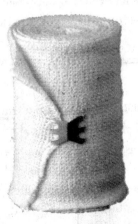

HERE ARE SOME BASIC SUPPLIES EVERY FIRST AID KIT SHOULD STOCK. OTHERWISE, THE AMOUNT AND TYPE OF ITEMS TO STOCK DEPENDS ON THE NEEDS OF YOUR SITE OR ACTIVITY, PORTABILITY, AND THE NUMBER OF PEOPLE INVOLVED.

Workplace
- Local guidelines and legislation dictate kit requirements.
- Learn where the first aid kits are located.

Home and car
- Clearly label the kit "First Aid." Show everyone where to find the kit – at home this might be a designated shelf in the medicine cabinet or a basket in a closet.
- Establish a routine for keeping it stocked. Keep a list of contents in the kit and restock it immediately after using any supplies.
- Organize it so it is easy to use in an emergency.
- Containers: If possible, choose a bright colour and something that is water resistant (e.g. plastic food containers, sealable food bags, fanny packs, recycled tins or jars).

Recommended contents

Dressings and bandages
- assorted bandage strips, rolls of adhesive tape, gauze pads
- compress dressings or cloth triangular bandages
- eye dressings

Equipment
- tweezers
- scissors
- barrier devices: pocket mask for rescue breathing, gloves
- safety pins (assorted sizes)
- splints and splint padding
- instant heat and cold packs
- waterproof waste bag
- EMS phone number(s)
- pencil and paper
- thermometer
- sterile saline solution (or bottle of water)

Other equipment (adapt the contents of the kit to suit your situation)
- waterproof matches
- pocket knife, penlight, whistle
- blanket (in the car)

Prevention of disease

In many rescues you may come into contact with fluids from the victim's body – mainly blood, vomit or spittle – with the potential to spread communicable diseases.

Although intact skin provides an effective barrier, medical evidence suggests that cross-contamination may result from mouth-to-mouth, hand-to-mouth, hand-to-eye or hand-to-nose contact. Cross-contamination means germs cross between the victim and the rescuer in either direction.

Protection

Gloves: Wear disposable gloves to create a barrier between you and any fluids. Prepare ahead by putting them on as you approach an emergency scene. If they tear at any time, replace them right away, and use clean gloves for each victim. Store gloves at room temperature and avoid leaving them in extreme heat or cold.

Removing gloves: Avoid spreading potential contaminants when removing used gloves. Whether they appear soiled or not, take them off inside-out, placing one inside the other:

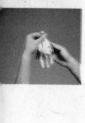

- Start by peeling one glove up over your fingers so it is inside out.
- Use the gloved hand to catch and hold the glove.
- Peel the second glove off in the same way, starting under the cuff to avoid touching the outside surface.
- As you peel, trap the first glove inside the second.
- Dispose of the gloves by placing them in another plastic bag, tie it and put it in your regular garbage.

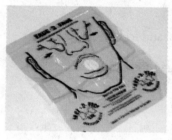 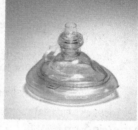

face shield   **pocket mask**

Rescue breathing devices: Although a barrier device is any object or ventilation system that provides some protection against cross-contamination, it primarily refers to devices used during rescue breathing. One of the simplest devices is a **face shield**, which is placed between the mouths of the victim and rescuer. Another common device is a **pocket mask**, usually equipped with a one-way valve to allow the rescuer to blow air into the victim, while directing exhaled air through vents away from the rescuer.

Each barrier device is different, so read and follow the manufacturer's directions for use and care. Barrier devices are disposable and should be thrown out when contaminated. During training you may use a barrier device more than once, but do not share it with others.

Wash your hands: Washing with warm water and soap will always be a practical way to help prevent disease. Liquid soap is preferred; lather for at least 1–2 minutes, rinse and dry thoroughly. Do this as soon as possible after performing a rescue or administering first aid, even if you were wearing gloves.

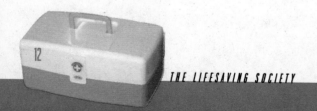

CRITICAL INCIDENT STRESS

FIRST AIDERS NEED TO RECOGNIZE THAT EMERGENCIES ARE INHERENTLY STRESSFUL AND NOT ALL OUTCOMES ARE SUCCESSFUL. WHEN THE INCIDENT IS OVER YOU GENERALLY FEEL RELIEF, THOUGH YOU MAY ALSO EXPERIENCE IMMEDIATE OR LINGERING FEELINGS OF GUILT OR SELF-DOUBT. THIS IS NORMAL. WHEN THESE REACTIONS INTERFERE WITH THE ABILITY TO FUNCTION DURING OR AFTER THE EMERGENCY, THEY ARE REFERRED TO AS CRITICAL INCIDENT STRESS (CIS) SYNDROME.

Signs & symptoms

Delayed CIS

- increasing feelings of depression, anxiety, and irritability
- sleep disturbance
- changes in eating habits
- loss of emotional control
- feelings of isolation
- disturbances of the menstrual cycle
- increased problems with interpersonal relations
- disturbing memories
- fear of repetition of the incident

Acute CIS

Physical
- nausea, sweating, tremors
- disorientation, loss of coordination
- increased heart rate and blood pressure
- hyperventilation, with chest pains and headaches
- muscle soreness
- difficulty sleeping, fatigue

Mental
- impaired thinking and decision making
- poor concentration, confusion, difficulty performing simple mental tasks
- difficulty with tasks involving memory
- flashbacks

Emotional
- anxiety, fear, guilt
- grief, depression
- emotional numbness
- feeling lost, abandoned, helpless
- withdrawal from others
- anger, resentment, blaming others
- feeling overwhelmed

Treatment

Do:
- Remember, it's natural for the incident to bother you.
- Maintain a healthy lifestyle – follow a good diet, exercise, and take time for leisure activities.
- Remind yourself that your reactions are normal.
- Learn as much as you can about critical incident stress syndrome.
- Spend time with family, friends and coworkers.
- Talk about it – find someone you're comfortable with and share your feelings about the incident.
- Realize that it can take months or years to deal with all aspects of the incident.
- Get professional help if necessary.

Don't:
- Deny or suppress your feelings by drinking or taking drugs.
- Withdraw from family, friends and coworkers.
- Avoid work.
- Use off-duty time for training immediately after the incident.
- Look for easy answers to explain why the incident happened.
- Think you are crazy, or that something is wrong with you.
- Have unrealistic expectations for recovery.

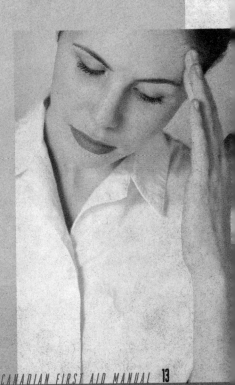

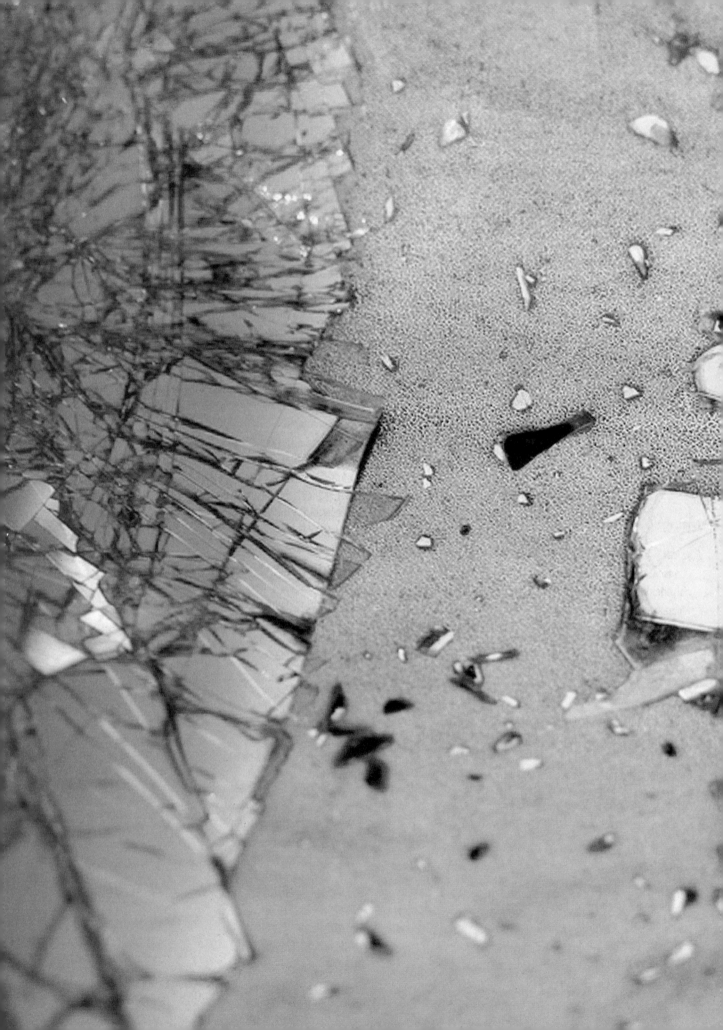

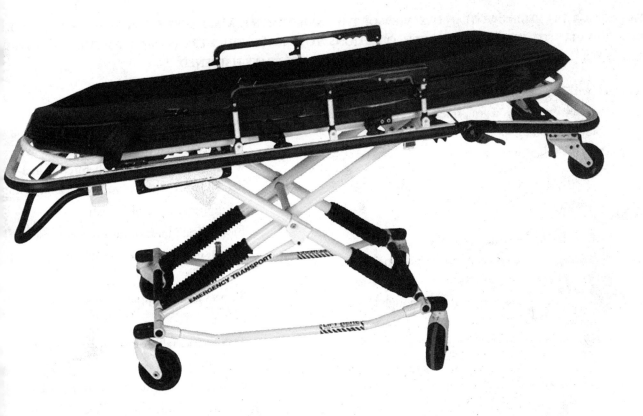

THE SCENE

RECOGNITION

A TYPICAL FIRST AID EMERGENCY OCCURS WITHOUT NOTICE, WHEN YOU LEAST EXPECT IT. IF THERE ARE PEOPLE AT THE SCENE, CONFUSION MAY ENSUE AS PEOPLE SCRAMBLE TO DECIDE WHAT TO DO. YOUR ABILITY TO RECOGNIZE SOMEONE IN TROUBLE WHO NEEDS HELP, AND REACT APPROPRIATELY, IS ESSENTIAL TO EFFECTIVE ACTION IN A FIRST AID EMERGENCY.

SCENE ASSESSMENT

A SCENE ASSESSMENT BEGINS WITH AN OVERVIEW OF THE ENVIRONMENT. MAKE SURE IT IS SAFE TO PROCEED, GET AN IDEA OF WHAT TO EXPECT AND WHICH QUESTIONS TO ASK. IF YOU WERE PRESENT AS THE EMERGENCY UNFOLDED YOU LIKELY HAVE A HEAD START BECAUSE YOU KNOW WHAT HAPPENED.

Approach with care and keep all of your senses open – rely on what you feel, smell, hear and see. Stay calm and respond methodically. Ask yourself the following questions.

Is it safe?

- Check for hazards such as a fallen ladder, broken glass, spilled chemicals or poisons, electrical appliances or traffic.
- What is the risk to you? Is it safe enough to enter the scene?
- Is the victim at risk of further harm?

What happened?

- Determine the mechanism of injury. Look for exactly what caused the injury. What was the victim doing just before the incident? Decide whether you are dealing with:
  a) injuries as a result of external forces
  b) medical illness or disorder as a result of unknown internal conditions

- Suspect a spinal injury if there was:
  a) a fall
  b) a considerable blow to the head, neck or back
  c) an obvious injury to the head or face
  d) if the victim is unconscious, confused or intoxicated and one of the above has occurred

Who is here?

- How many victims are present? Which onlookers can help you?

Change of scene?

- Monitor the environment, the victim and yourself. If the conditions of the surroundings change, the condition of the victim changes, or there is a change in the way you react or feel, it may require adjustments in treatment.

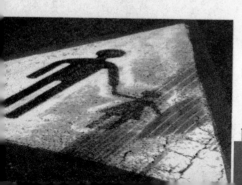

Call for help and attract attention

If you are not sure what you can do, or if you think the environment could put you in danger, get help from EMS or from bystanders.

Remove hazards

Ensure the area is safe by removing any hazards from the rescue environment or by removing the victim from the hazardous area. Separate yourself and the victim from any immediate or recurrent danger.

Multiple victims

When there is more than one victim, emphasis is placed on doing the most good for the greatest number. Therefore, treat victims with the most serious life-threatening injuries first, such as respiratory arrest or major bleeding.

First, conduct a primary assessment on all victims and immediately contact EMS if any victim is unresponsive or distressed. If you are treating multiple victims with life-threatening injuries, and cannot recruit enough help to treat them all, those with no signs of circulation are the lowest priority for treatment.

Proceed to secondary assessment only after you've dealt with the ABC priorities for all victims.

Multiple injuries

Focus on the ABC priorities and what you know how to do.

Spinal injuries

If you suspect a spinal injury, treat the victim as if there is a spinal injury. Do not move the victim (as far as conditions allow). Prevent movement by asking a bystander to hold the victim's head and neck still. If you are alone, use available objects to support the position of the victim.

Preliminaries

Make contact with the victim:

1. Say "hello" and introduce yourself.
2. Assure them of your skills and experience as a first aider.
3. Ask if you can help – you must obtain the victim's consent before continuing.
4. Learn and use the victim's name.
5. Start reassuring victim immediately.

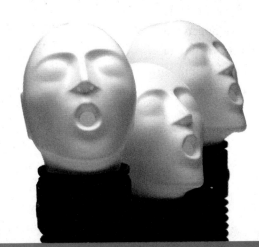

PRIMARY EMERGENCIES

RECOGNITION: ABC PRIORITIES

Unless specifically noted, the techniques described in this book are for adults. The ages listed below are only guidelines – always consider the victim's size as well.

Adult	**8 years and over**
Child	**1 to 8 years**
Infant	**birth to 1 year**

ONCE THE FIRST AIDER COMPLETES A SCENE ASSESSMENT AND TAKES ACTION TO ELIMINATE LIFE-THREATENING CONDITIONS IN THE ENVIRONMENT, HE OR SHE CAN TEND TO THE "CASUALTIES" OR "VICTIMS."

Life-threatening conditions

The first priority of a first aider is to treat life-threatening conditions. The most urgent life-threatening conditions occur when breathing stops, when the blood stops circulating or the heart ceases to beat. Then, look for those who still have these functions, but may be in danger of slipping into a life-threatening state in the next few minutes. These emergencies are classified as "ABC Priorities," i.e., anything that affects consciousness and the quality of breathing and circulation, including shock and major bleeding.

Recognizing a breathing emergency

Breathing difficulties are classified in three major categories:

1. *Reduced oxygen* – poisonous gas, smoke, suffocation (something blocking the nose and mouth), drowning
2. *Airway obstructions/choking* – tongue, water, foreign objects, strangulation (something around the outside of the neck or throat)
3. *Malfunctions of the heart and lung caused by:*
   a) interference in the brain – head or spinal injuries, poisonous drugs, heart attack, electric shock, low blood sugar
   b) injuries to the respiratory system – airway, lungs, diaphragm

Permanent brain damage may result if a person goes without oxygen for more than four minutes.

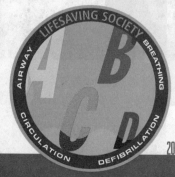

PRIMARY ASSESSMENT

THE PRIMARY ASSESSMENT DETERMINES IF LIFE-THREATENING CONDITIONS EXIST.
IT ASKS "YES" OR "NO" QUESTIONS.

Assess		Question
LOC	Level of consciousness	Is the victim responsive and conscious?
A	Airway	Is the airway open?
B	Breathing	Is the victim breathing normally?
C	Circulation	Is blood circulating sufficiently throughout the body?

Where the answer is "yes"

The primary assessment is virtually unnoticed. The victim is responsive and can speak freely and coherently. Rescuers proceed to the secondary assessment.

Where the answer is "no"

When there is no response, ineffective breathing, and no signs of circulation or evidence of major bleeding, the primary assessment flows seamlessly into treatment of these emergencies. The rescuer must phone EMS immediately and treat the symptoms.

Decision Flow Chart

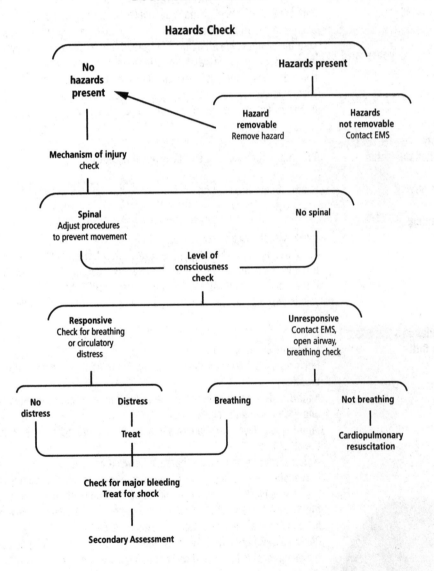

ACTION: ABC PRIORITIES

Sequence of steps

The following sequence includes both assessment and treatment. It assumes the worst-case scenario – the victim has no circulation. Depending on your assessment, you may exit this sequence and move to treat less severe breathing and circulatory emergencies, or move to secondary assessment and treatment.

Reminder: Complete a scene assessment first, which includes determining whether to treat for a suspected spinal injury.

Step	Action
Level of consciousness (LOC)	
Establish unresponsiveness	☐ Gently squeeze or pinch shoulders; ask "Are you OK?" ☐ A victim is unresponsive if there is no verbal answer or no movement in response to the squeeze or pinch.
Phone EMS	☐ Activate EMS. If no cellphone is available, send a bystander to call EMS and get an AED if possible. If you're alone with an adult victim, you'll have to go make the call yourself. If you are alone with a child or infant, make sure the victim is breathing or, if not breathing, perform about 5 cycles (about 2 minutes) of CPR (30:2 compressions: breaths) before leaving the victim to phone EMS. ☐ If you are alone and must leave the unconscious victim, carefully place the victim in the recovery position to ensure airway drainage (assuming you do not suspect a spinal injury). It is often possible to carry a child or infant victim while ensuring a drainage position. If so, carry them to the telephone with you and call EMS.
Airway	
Position the victim	☐ Turn the victim over to open the airway if necessary.
Open airway	☐ Head-tilt/chin-lift. With an unconscious victim, always assume the airway is blocked by the tongue.
Breathing	
Look	☐ Quick, visual check (5 sec.). ☐ Kneel beside victim. Maintain open airway. Watch the victim's chest and abdomen for breathing movements. ☐ If the victim is breathing, place in recovery position and monitor breathing. ☐ If the victim is not breathing, start CPR. Begin CPR on an unresponsive adult who is not breathing normally or who is gasping. An unresponsive, gasping adult victim is probably in cardiac arrest and requires CPR.
Circulation	
Start CPR	☐ Landmark on victim's chest. ☐ **Perform chest compressions** (count out loud): Adult, child and infant – sets of 30 compressions with 2 breaths. ☐ Adult/Child – seal mouth, pinch nose. Give 2 normal (not deep) breaths – each breath delivered over 1 second and each making the chest rise. ☐ Infant – seal over baby's mouth and nose, blow gentle puffs. Give 2 normal (not deep) breaths – each making the chest rise. ☐ Watch chest rise and allow exhalation between breaths. ☐ If available, use barrier devices – position barrier device over victim's mouth and nose. ☐ If airway is blocked, treat as an unconscious victim with an obstructed airway. ☐ Child and infant victims – after about 5 cycles of 30:2 compressions:breaths, phone EMS if you are alone or have not already sent a bystander to make the call. ☐ Continue CPR until EMS takes over treatment, or an AED-trained responder begins treatment with AED unit, or the victim begins to move. If the victim begins to move, reassess ABCs and treat appropriately.

Step	Action

Two-rescuer CPR

When two rescuers are first at the scene: Assess the scene, phone EMS (or get someone else to make the call). One rescuer (compressor) does chest compressions while the second rescuer (ventilator) performs rescue breathing. Rescuers communicate and cooperate in decision-making and in performing CPR.

Fatigue can begin to affect the effectiveness of compressions in as little as 2 minutes. Two-rescuer CPR minimizes fatigue by allowing rescuers to take turns doing compressions, changing about every 5 cycles of 30:2 (about 2 minutes).

To switch positions, the compressor says "Switch" after performing compressions and moves beside the victim's head to become the ventilator. The new compressor changes position, landmarks and begins compressions. Rescuers should minimize the time it takes to switch positions – less than 10 seconds.

When one rescuer joins a scene where CPR is already started: He or she indicates knowledge of CPR and checks to make sure EMS is activated, then offers to help with CPR.

When two rescuers arrive at a scene where one rescuer is already performing CPR:
Try to take over without interrupting CPR. Identify yourself as first aiders and suggest you'll take over after two breaths. The ventilator assesses the victim and the compressor moves into position. Begin two-person CPR.

Each rescuer may also take turns doing one rescuer CPR.

If victim is breathing and has circulation:

Check for major bleeding
- Do a quick visual check.
- Wear gloves.
- Complete a quick hands-on inspection of the victim from head-to-toe in case blood is pooling out of sight. Make sure your hands go under all natural body hollows (e.g. small of the back, behind the knees) and then look for blood on your gloves. (If the victim is conscious or semi-conscious, describe what you are doing.)

Treat for shock
Assume shock is present in any injury or illness.

Next:
- If the victim is breathing, unconscious and shows no signs of spinal injury, place in recovery position.
- If the victim is breathing, but shows signs of other ABC emergencies, treat those emergencies.
- Once all ABC emergencies are treated, move to secondary assessment and treatment.

CPR AND DROWNING VICTIMS

The primary cause of death from drowning is suffocation – a lack of oxygen. A drowning victim requires oxygen fast. The first and most important treatment is the immediate provision of ventilation. Start CPR with 2 rescue breaths followed by compressions.

PULSE CHECKS

The 2005 CPR Guidelines removed pulse checks by first aiders during primary assessments. The research showed that first aiders and health care providers alike had difficulty accurately assessing pulse in an unresponsive non-breathing victim. And this resulted in delay in performing CPR. First aiders should assume that cardiac arrest is present if the unresponsive victim is not breathing.

"LIFE OVER LIMB"

If treating a life-threatening injury aggravates another injury (or suspected injury), the need to tend to "life" (airway, breathing and circulation) takes priority over a secondary injury, "limb." For example, it may be necessary to move a spinal-injured victim without adequate immobilization in order to perform CPR.

NOTES ON TECHNIQUES FOR PRIMARY ASSESSMENT

To open an airway

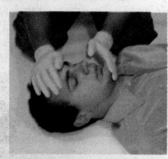

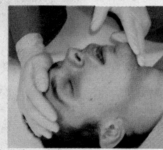

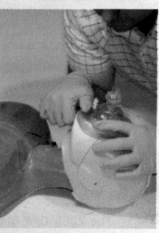

Head-tilt/chin-lift. Kneel beside the victim's head and open the airway. If the victim is an adult:

- Using your hand that is closest to the victim's head, place it on the forehead and apply firm backward (downward) pressure with your palm to tilt the head back.
- Place the first two fingers of your other hand under the bony part of the victim's lower jaw, near the chin. Lift to bring the chin forward (upward) and almost close the teeth.
- Maintain pressure on the chin, both up and towards the forehead, so the bottom of the ear lobe and the chin form a straight line at right angles to the floor.

If the victim is a child or infant, be careful not to overextend the neck.

Jaw thrust

- If a spinal injury is suspected, grasp the victim's jaw on both sides of the face where it forms an angle close to the ears. Using both hands, move the jaw forward (upward) without tilting the head back. Unless using a pocket mask, seal the victim's nose with your thumbs or cheek while performing rescue breaths.

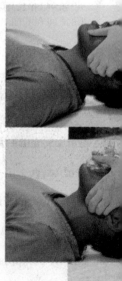

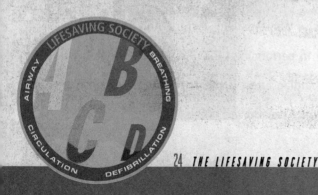

Special rescue breathing techniques

When mouth-to-mouth rescue breathing is not possible because of injury to the victim's mouth or previous surgery, use one of the following:

Mouth-to-nose: When it is not possible to seal the victim's mouth, try mouth-to-nose rescue breathing. Close the victim's mouth and seal your mouth around the victim's nose. Give two full breaths and observe the chest rise to ensure the air goes in.

Mouth-to-stoma: Some people have surgery to remove part of their trachea (windpipe). They breathe through a hole called a stoma in the front of the neck. Hold the mouth and nose closed and perform rescue breathing using the stoma. Watch to see that the chest rises to ensure the air goes in.

Foreign matter obstruction

When the upper airway is obstructed by foreign matter or an object, remove it with sweeps of the finger. If this proves difficult, turn the victim to his or her side and remove the object from the mouth and throat. Foreign objects may include dentures, gum, food, broken teeth, blood, toys, food, or plant debris if the victim is in the water.

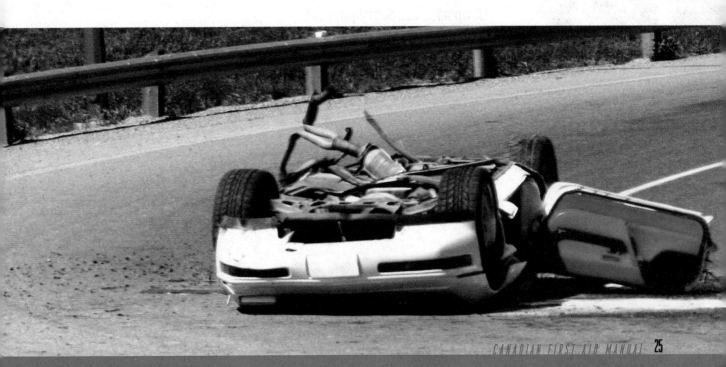

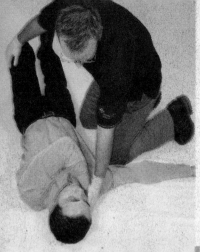

Recovery positions

If a spinal injury isn't suspected, place a breathing unconscious victim in the recovery (semi-prone) position. This is a stable position that helps maintain an open airway and allows fluids to drain down and out. It still permits you to check vital signs and conduct a head-to-toe examination for the secondary assessment.

How to roll from back to recovery: Protect the heads of victims when moving them into the recovery position. Follow these steps:

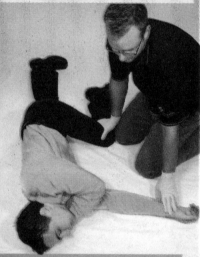

1. Put the arm nearest to you straight out, perpendicular to the body. If the victim is too heavy to roll, put the arm parallel to the body directly above the head.

2. Hold the palm of the farthest arm, pull the arm, bend it and place it under the victim's neck or ear.

3. Bend the knee of the far leg so it points up.

4. Roll the victim by pulling the bent knee towards you, over the near leg and to the ground. Protect the head while rolling. Rest the leg on the ground to stabilize the lower body.

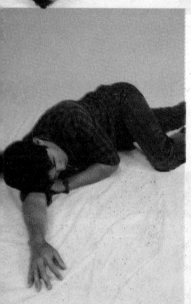

5. Adjust the hand supporting the neck and the position of the arms and legs so the victim is in a stable position. Adjust the shoulder so it rests relatively flat against the floor.

Alternate recovery position

In this alternative recovery position, the head rests on the extended arm and remains in line with the spine.

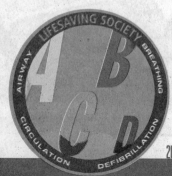

Cardiopulmonary Resuscitation (CPR)

CPR IS A COMBINATION OF TWO LIFE SUPPORT TECHNIQUES:

1. **ARTIFICIAL RESPIRATION** – BLOWING AIR INTO THE LUNGS.

2. **ARTIFICIAL CIRCULATION** – PUMPING THE CHEST TO CIRCULATE OXYGENATED BLOOD THROUGHOUT THE BODY.

Landmarking

The purpose of landmarking is to target compressions to the most effective area of the chest without causing injury, such as breaking the tip of the breastbone. Practice landmarking on real people, but do not apply pressure during practice.

There are a variety of landmarking methods. Try these:

- **Adult and child:** place hands on centre of chest. Landmark on the centre of a line drawn between the nipples and position both hands on the sternum, one hand on top of the other for vertical compressions. Keep elbows locked straight during compressions.
- **Infant:** landmark one finger width below the centre of the nipple line and use two fingers for compressions.

Chest compressions

Compressions squeeze the heart between the breastbone and the backbones. This action artificially pumps enough blood and oxygen to the body to sustain vital organs. The goal is to compress straight down from the breastbone towards the backbone. Two things help you avoid pushing sideways at an angle:

1. Positioning hands for vertical compressions:

- **Adults:** Landmark, then interlace your fingers and lift them off the ribs so you are only using the heels of your hands.
- **Children:** The rescuer can perform compressions using one or two hands. One-hand technique is shown in the picture below.
- **Infants:** Use two fingers to perform compressions.

Depth: How far to push down the breastbone

- **Adult:** At least 5 cm (2 in.) but no more than 6 cm (2.4 in.)
- **Child:** at least 1/3 chest diameter or 5 cm (2 in.)
- **Infant:** at least 1/3 chest diameter or 4 cm (1 1/2 in.)

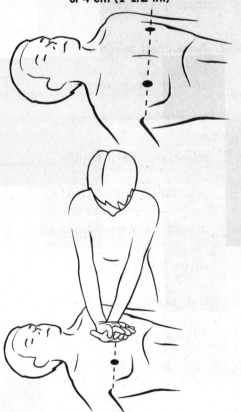

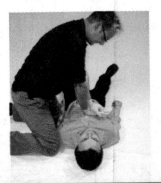

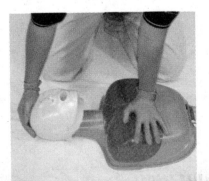

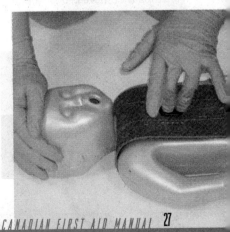

Three tips for good, effective CPR

1. **Push hard and fast** (100/min. to 120/min.). Forceful, fast CPR provides better circulation of blood and oxygen.

2. **Allow chest to recoil fully** between compressions: 50% compression, 50% relaxation. Relaxing the pressure on the chest between compressions allows the heart to refill and pump more blood with each compression.

3. **Minimize interruptions** in compressions. Blood flow stops if compressions stop.

2. Keep elbows locked straight (Adult and Child):

- Start by landmarking with your shoulders directly over the victim's breastbone.
- Then look up and straight ahead.
- Rock your upper body into the compression using your weight to press down instead of only using your arm muscles.

Counting: You are not counting seconds: count "1-and," not "1-1000" or "1-Mississippi." Count "1" on the down stroke and "and" on the upstroke to keep it smooth. Do not move your hands out of position, simply apply and release pressure.

Aim for a minimum of 100 compressions per minute to a maximum of 120 compressions per minute, or just under two compressions per second. This means 30 compressions in 15 to 18 seconds. Track the number of cycles by counting when you do the ventilations. If you get lost in all the counting, don't worry; keep performing chest compressions to the best of your ability.

CPR with pregnant victims: Put a pillow or some wedge-shaped object under the right side of the woman's abdomen. This shifts the uterus to the left side and helps blood return to the heart.

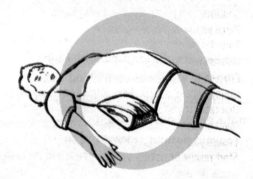

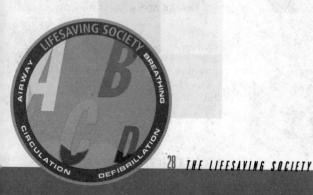

Rescue breathing complications

If this is present...	then do this:
Victim vomits	Roll victim on side. (Turning the victim towards you allows easy access to the mouth.) Allow vomit to drain and finger sweep to clear the mouth. Resume rescue breathing.
Gastric distension (stomach expands instead of the chest)	Blowing too hard or quickly may send air into the stomach causing it to swell. This makes it harder to perform rescue breathing and increases the chance of the victim vomiting. If you notice gastric distension: Reposition the head; make sure it is tilted back enough so the airway is completely open. Deliver each breath (not deep) over 1 second. Each breath should make the chest rise. Watch the chest rise and allow exhalation between breaths. Blow just enough air to make the chest rise.
It is not possible to seal the victim's mouth	Perform mouth-to-nose rescue breathing. Close the mouth and make the seal with your mouth around the victim's nose. (Don't pinch the nose.)
The victim breathes through a stoma (a surgical hole in the victim's neck)	Perform mouth-to-stoma rescue breathing. Close the mouth and pinch the nose. Seal your mouth around the victim's stoma.
Ineffective breathing (low rate of respiration, or slow breathing)	Assisted breathing: Effective breathing means breathing normally. When breathing is ineffective, the body may not be getting enough oxygen to function. Begin assisted breathing as soon as you recognize any signs of severe breathing difficulty in conscious or unconscious victims. If the victim is conscious, explain what you are doing. The technique is to use standard rescue breathing with modified timing of ventilations: If the victim is unconscious and breathing too slow: Give a breath each time the victim inhales plus one extra breath in between. Give a breath every 5 seconds for a total of 12–15 breaths per minute. If the victim is unconscious and breathing too fast: Give a breath on every second inhalation for a total of 12–15 breaths per minute.
Victim begins to breathe without assistance	Continue to monitor ABCs and vital signs. Place victim in recovery position. Treat for shock. Be prepared to begin rescue breathing again. Proceed to secondary assessment.
You become physically tired **Two rescuers**	Change operators, i.e., have a bystander take over for you. One rescuer performs rescue breathing (you may change operators). Another rescuer proceeds with the secondary assessment.
Victim is in the water	Ensure your own safety and that of the victim. Start rescue breathing as soon as you and the victim are in shallow water where you can comfortably check the airway. When you are doing rescue breathing in the water, use the head-tilt manoeuvre to open the airway. That is, using your arm closest to the victim's feet, place it between the near arm and the victim's torso. Then, press the back of your hand against the victim's spine at the bottom the neck or between the shoulder blades. Lift the upper body. The chest will rise, the head will fall back to extend the neck and the rest of the body will be somewhat vertical. The body will still float keeping most of the victim's weight in the water. Keep the victim's nose pinched throughout rescue breathing. Get out of cold water as soon as possible. Strong currents make it harder to control the victim. So move away from them, or work with currents, not against them.

ACTION: OTHER BREATHING EMERGENCIES

Obstructed airways – Choking

The tongue is the most common cause of an airway obstruction in an unconscious victim. This is why "A – open the airway" is the first priority. Other causes for choking are blood from facial and head injuries, vomit, severe allergic reaction, infection, food and other foreign objects. In every case, act promptly to relieve the blockage before the victim becomes unconscious.

Adults: Choking in the conscious adult is most often caused by large poorly chewed pieces of food. Dentures and alcohol intoxication are also common factors.

Children: Since children have a tendency to put small objects or toys into their mouths, supervision and prevention are the best deterrents:

- Supervise children when they are playing with balloons and other small toys.
- Check your house regularly for small objects.

- Always supervise children while they eat and teach them not to move around while eating.
- Cut food into manageable pieces and don't feed small items to young kids such as nuts, popcorn, small candies or thick peanut butter.

Infants: Infants are also likely to put small objects or toys into their mouths. To prevent infant breathing emergencies:

- Supervise them as they eat and feed them small pieces of food.
- Inspect their toys for small removable parts and keep toys out of their crib.
- Do not let them play with balloons or other small toys involving the mouth.
- Check pacifiers for worn nipples.

Severe or mild obstructions: A severe obstruction does not allow the air to pass by the object. A mild obstruction allows some air to pass, yet it can still be very distressing.

Airway obstruction procedures – conscious and unconscious

Signs and symptoms	Treatment
Conscious victim	
	☐ Approach, identify yourself. If a choking victim leaves the room, follow.
	☐ Ask: "Are you choking? My name is… and I am trained in first aid. Can I help?"
Good air exchange:	☐ As long as a victim is coughing and clearing the airway on his or her own, do not interfere physically.
☐ coughing forcefully	☐ Monitor the situation. If the victim leaves the room, follow. The situation may deteriorate.
☐ can speak	
☐ wheezing between coughs	
☐ flushed skin colour	

Note: If you are the one choking, get the attention of people around you by holding your throat – the universal sign for choking. If you are alone, and your airway is completely obstructed, try giving yourself abdominal thrusts. Alternatively, you might try producing abdominal thrusts by pressing forcefully against the edge of a desk, counter top or other solid object.

Adult, child and infant –
severe obstructions:
- weak, ineffective cough
- cannot speak or cry
- may be holding the throat
- difficulty breathing
- no breathing noise
- grey/blue colour of the lips and gums

- Shout for help. Send a bystander to phone EMS.
- Reassure victim.

Adult and Child
- Back blows, abdominal thrusts or chest thrusts are effective for relieving severe airway obstruction in conscious adults and children. These techniques (see page 32) should be applied in rapid sequence until the obstruction is relieved or the victim becomes unconscious. More than one technique may be needed; there is insufficient evidence to determine which should be used first.
- Some jurisdictions follow a standardized protocol. E.g., for Emergency or Standard First Aid certification in Ontario, 5 back blows alternate with 5 abdominal thrusts.

Infant
- Perform 5 back blows.
- Perform 5 chest compressions.
- Repeat until successful or victim becomes unconscious.

If victim is pregnant or too
large for you to deliver
abdominal thrusts
- Perform chest compressions instead of abdominal thrusts.
- Landmark the same as in CPR compressions.
- Pull straight back, not in an upward motion.

If the victim becomes
unconscious

Adult and Child
- Assist the victim to the floor to prevent injury.
- Phone EMS. (Send a bystander if one is available.)
- Perform 30 compressions.
- Open mouth: check for foreign object – if you see it, remove it.
- Give a breath: if air goes in, give another breath. If air does not go in, reposition head and try again.
- Continue compressions and breaths until victim responds or EMS arrives.

Infant
- Phone EMS. (Send a bystander, or if you make the call yourself, take the infant with you.)
- Perform 30 compressions.
- Open mouth: check for foreign object – if you see it remove it.
- Give a breath (a puff): if air goes in, give another puff. If air does not go in, reposition head and try again.
- Continue compressions and breaths until victim responds or EMS arrives.

Unconscious victim
- Phone EMS. (Send a bystander if one is available.)

Primary assessment:
- air does not enter when attempting to ventilate

Adult, Child and Infant
- Open airway: check for breathing. Start CPR if not breathing or not breathing normally.
- Perform 30 compressions.
- Give a breath: if air goes in, give another breath. If air does not go in, reposition head and try again.
- Continue with another 30 compressions.
- Open mouth: check for foreign object – if you see it, remove it.
- Continue sequence of breaths, compressions and checks for foreign object until victim responds or EMS arrives.

Techniques for choking emergencies

Foreign object checks

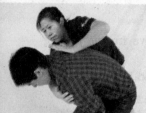

- Look inside the mouth for the obstruction. If you see it, remove it using a hooked finger by pulling it up against the near cheek – be careful, the object may be sharp or hard to handle.

Adult and child

Back blows:

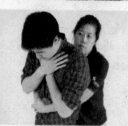

- Support the victim's chest with one arm. Bend the victim near parallel to the ground. Apply back blows with the palm of your free hand between the shoulder blades. If unsuccessful, continue with 5 abdominal thrusts.

Abdominal thrusts:

- Stand behind the victim and wrap your arms around his or her waist. Make a fist with one hand. Place the thumb side of the fist against the victim's abdomen in the midline, slightly above the navel and well below the soft lower tip of the breastbone. Grasp your fist with your other hand and press the fist into the victim's abdomen with a quick upward thrust. Each thrust should be a separate and distinct movement. Repeat the thrusts until the airway is clear. (Abdominal thrusts can be performed effectively while standing in shallow water.)

Chest compressions:

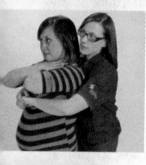

- Effective if the victim is too large for you to perform abdominal thrusts or if she is pregnant.
- Stand behind the victim and wrap your arms around his or her chest under the armpits. Grab your fist with the other hand and place the thumb side in the centre of the victim's breastbone. Press with quick backward thrusts.

Infant

Back blows:

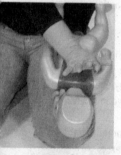

- Kneel or sit and brace supporting arm on thigh or lap. Position baby face down on supporting arm, head lower than the rest of the body. Support baby's head. When face down, hold baby's jaw. Deliver 5 back blows between the shoulder blades using the heel of the free hand.

Chest compressions:

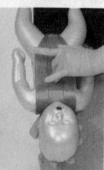

- Turn the baby over to a face-up position or transfer baby from one arm to the other. Deliver 5 chest compressions using the same technique and landmarking as for infant CPR. Use 2 fingers. Press straight down 1/3 depth of the chest.

Unconscious victims:

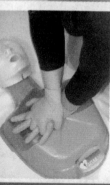

- Landmark as in CPR – on the centre of an imaginary line drawn between the nipples.
- Position hands and body for CPR compressions, push straight down:
  - Adult: 5 cm (2 in.)
  - Child and infant: 1/3 depth of chest

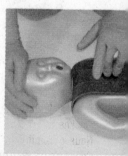

Asthma

Asthma is a breathing disorder in which airway sensitivity is increased. This sensitivity results in spasms of the airway muscles and increased production of mucus, which narrows the airway and blocks air exchange. Common triggers to an asthma attack include allergies, emotional distress and extreme temperatures.

Asthma – victim and incident history:
Check for medical condition identification and medication.

Signs and symptoms	Treatment
Difficulty breathing	Assist the victim to a comfortable position: while sitting or standing, try leaning forward slightly with the arms resting on some object.
Anxiety	Help the victim take his or her medication (e.g. inhaler). See p.44.
Wheezing	Loosen tight-fitting clothing around the neck or chest.
	If the asthma attack continues or the victim is distressed, arrange for transportation to hospital by contacting EMS.

Hyperventilation

When someone begins to breathe faster or deeper than necessary, it looks like "over-breathing" and is called hyperventilation. Hyperventilation reduces the level of carbon dioxide in the blood, which can depress the brain's breathing centre and result in unconsciousness.

Hyperventilation may be a reaction to fear or stress, or it may be brought on intentionally. Swimmers may hyperventilate in an effort to swim farther or deeper under the surface.

Treatment aims to increase the amount of carbon dioxide in the victim's blood, which allows normal breathing to return within a few minutes.

Hyperventilation – victim and incident history:
If hyperventilation has not happened before, watch for chest pain or other signs of heart attack or more serious medical problems.

Signs and symptoms	Treatment
High rate of respiration, panting, gasping	Reassure and try to calm victim.
Lightheadedness, weakness, headache	Phone EMS.
Tingling of hands, feet, and the area around the mouth	
Confusion, unconsciousness	

Drowning

Drowning victims can suffocate when the airway is blocked by water and insufficient oxygen reaches the blood and tissues. In some cases aspiration of water, dirt, bacteria, oils or detergents can damage the respiratory system. This complicates resuscitation and may negatively affect outcomes. Symptoms may be delayed up to 72 hours after the event.

Drowning

Signs and symptoms	Treatment
LOC: reduced level of consciousness	Advise a conscious victim to see a doctor. Give a warning about the seriousness of any later symptoms of respiratory distress.
Breathing: shallow or rapid	
Coughing or wheezing	Phone EMS if vital signs are abnormal or victim is distressed.
Anxiety	
Weakness	
Nausea, vomiting	
Coughing up whitish or pink frothy fluid	
Shock	

See p.44.

PURSED-LIP BREATHING

Asthmatics have trouble getting air out. Pursed-lip breathing is when the lips are in a "pucker" position and the victim blows air out in a slow, steady stream. You and the victim can do this together. Inhale through the nose, exhale through the pursed lips and focus on getting air out.

AIRWAY MANAGEMENT IN DROWNING VICTIMS

In most documented cases, airway management in drowning victims is a significant challenge. Be extremely attentive to clearing fluids. The amount of fluid and vomit that needs to be managed is often unexpected. You will need to place the victim in the recovery position to provide drainage and protect the airway.

RISK FACTORS FOR HEART DISEASE AND STROKE

In Canada, thousands of people die every year from heart disease and stroke. Half of these deaths occur before the victim reaches hospital.

Several factors directly increase the risk of heart disease or stroke. The three major factors are:

1. *Smoking* – the leading risk factor.

2. *High blood pressure* (hypertension) – high pressure within the blood vessels adds to the workload of the heart.

3. *High cholesterol* – deposits cause atherosclerosis; a narrowing of the arteries that increases the risk of blockage within the arteries of the heart and brain.

Some risk factors of heart disease cannot be changed, such as age, gender and heredity. But it is possible for a person to control risk factors such as body weight (obesity), smoking, blood pressure, exercise, cholesterol and stress.

Choosing a healthy lifestyle that includes regular exercise, eating a balanced diet, and regular check-ups with your doctor can significantly reduce your risk of heart disease. For more information about healthy choices and your risk factors, talk to your doctor or contact the *Heart and Stroke Foundation of Canada*.

ACTION: OTHER CIRCULATORY EMERGENCIES

Angina and heart attack

Angina and heart attack happen when the heart muscle does not receive enough blood and oxygen.

Angina, a medically diagnosed condition, is caused by poor blood circulation to the heart. Someone with heart disease may experience angina when under stress or while being more physically active than usual.

Heart attack occurs when a blood vessel carrying blood and oxygen to the heart is blocked. The severity of the heart attack, and the damage to the heart muscle, depend on the duration of the interruption in blood flow to the heart and the extent of the muscle affected.

Angina and heart attack – victim and incident history:
Check for medical condition identification and medication.

Signs and symptoms	Treatment
☐ Breathing: trouble breathing, shortness of breath	If known history of angina:
☐ Skin: flushed face, sweating	☐ Phone EMS.
	☐ Assist the victim into a comfortable position. This is often a semi-sitting position.
☐ Pain, pressure, or tightness in the chest or shoulder	☐ Loosen tight clothing around the neck and chest.
☐ Anxiety, fear, confusion	☐ Help a conscious victim take any prescribed angina medication. (See sidebar "Helping with Medication" p. 44.) Common medications for angina are nitroglycerin tablets or sprays.
☐ Shock	If the victim uses Viagra®, taking nitroglycerin may cause a significant decrease in blood pressure.
☐ Circulation: weak, rapid pulse	☐ If the victim does not have prescribed medication, another option is ASA. First, confirm the victim is not allergic to ASA, and hasn't been told by a doctor to avoid ASA. Recommend the victim chew 1 adult or 2 low dose ASA tablets. The victim must choose whether or not to take medication. ASA can also reduce the effects of a heart attack.
☐ Pain in the arms, neck, back or jaw	
☐ Nausea, vomiting	
☐ Weakness, dizziness	☐ Do not substitute acetaminophen (Tylenol®) or ibuprofen (Advil®) for ASA.
☐ Fatigue	
☐ Indigestion	
☐ Denial of symptoms	If no history of angina and victim is distressed or shows symptoms not relieved by medication – phone EMS.

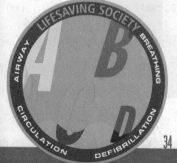

Stroke

A stroke occurs when the brain does not receive enough blood and oxygen due to internal bleeding or a blockage in a blood artery. Without blood, brain damage occurs and shows up in the victim as various sudden impairments.

Some stroke victims recover some function, and medical research has developed early intervention techniques that allow some patients to fully recover. But most live on with a physical or mental disability, or both. It is essential that stroke victims go to the hospital immediately after noticing the symptoms.

There are two causes of stroke:

1. A blockage in a brain artery.
2. An artery in the brain bursts and bleeds.

Stroke

Signs and symptoms	Treatment
☐ Weakness, numbness or tingling in the face, arm or leg	☐ Phone EMS.
☐ Facial droop	☐ Maintain an open airway.
☐ Sudden trouble speaking or understanding speech	☐ Assess breathing, check pulse and other signs of circulation.
☐ Double vision, sudden dimness or loss of vision, especially in one eye	☐ Assist the victim to a comfortable position (often semi-sitting) or a recovery position if there are airway management problems.
☐ Sudden, severe and unusual headache	
☐ Unexplained dizziness, unsteadiness	
☐ Unexplained loss of consciousness	
☐ See F.A.S.T sidebar	

Shock

Shock is a depression of the body's circulatory system. When there is not enough blood to circulate to the body's vital tissues (in the brain, heart and lungs), cells die – and ultimately, so can the victim.

Causes include:

- **Weak heart action, heart attack** – because the heart has been weakened by lack of oxygen, clogged arteries, or weak heart muscles.
- **Expansion of blood vessels** – in response to injury or some poisons, or severe allergic reactions affecting breathing and heart function.
- **Loss of blood and body** fluids – due to internal or external bleeding, severe burns and severe dehydration.
- **Spinal cord or nerve injuries**

Shock can be mild, with few signs and symptoms, or very serious with life-threatening signs and symptoms. The extent of shock is usually related to the severity of the injury to the body.

CARDIAC ARREST

Cardiac arrest is the term to describe the heart when it ceases to beat. It is usually caused by malfunctions of the heart and lung or in instances where there is reduced oxygen. Signs of cardiac arrest are unconsciousness, no pulse and no signs of circulation including breathing, coughing or movement in response to rescue breathing.

TRANSIENT ISCHEMIC ATTACK (TIA)

TIA is often a warning sign that the victim is at risk for a stroke. Five per cent of people with a TIA will develop a stroke within one month if untreated. Signs and symptoms are the same as for a stroke, but usually last for less than 20 minutes. Fast recognition and medical treatment may prevent stroke or reduce the amount of permanent damage.

F.A.S.T.

Use the acronym F.A.S.T. (Face. Arms. Speech. Time.) to help assess a suspected stroke victim. Is their **Face** drooping? Ask if they can smile. Is one arm weak or numb? Ask if they can raise one or both **Arms**. Does one arm drift downward? Is their **Speech** slurred or impaired? Ask if they can repeat a simple sentence. If you notice any of these signs do not delay. It is **Time** to act: call EMS.

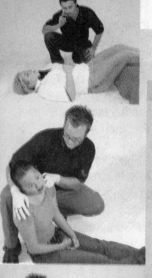

Shock – victim and incident history:
Assume that shock is present. Most injuries are accompanied by some degree of shock.

Signs and symptoms
- Breathing: shallow, rapid
- Circulation: weak, rapid pulse
- Skin: pale, cool, clammy
- Restlessness, weakness
- Fear, anxiety
- Confusion, disorientation
- Nausea, vomiting
- Unconsciousness

Treatment
Treat for shock as early as is practical, and only stop when you stop all first aid care.

The way to remember treatment for shock is the word **WARTS**:
- **Warmth**: Maintain body temperature. If the victim is in the sun, provide shade. If the victim's body is cool, cover the victim (put something under and over the victim).
- **ABCs**: Loosen tight clothing. Monitor vital signs.
- **Rest and reassurance**: Reassure the victim, and make sure he or she rests. Talk calmly, positively, and good-naturedly to the victim. Make eye contact when you speak and use a gentle, confident touch. Stay calm – your ability to cope with stress directly affects the victim and that's your priority.
- **Treatment**: Treat the cause of the shock (e.g. a wound or heart attack).
- **Semi-prone (recovery) position**: Use this position when you don't suspect a head or spinal injury and the victim is less than fully conscious. If the victim is fully conscious (and you don't suspect a head or spinal injury) the **shock position** is to place the victim on his or her back with the feet and legs raised. If you do suspect a head or spinal injury, keep the victim in the **position found** to prevent further injury. A **semi-sitting** position is recommended for chest pain or shortness of breath. Ultimately, you want the victim in a position where he or she is most comfortable, and usually the injury or illness will dictate the best position.
- Phone EMS.

Major bleeding

Severe bleeding is an ABC emergency because of its connection to "C – the circulatory system."

Major bleeding

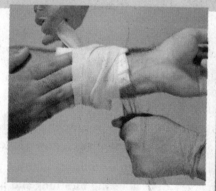

Signs and symptoms
- Blood
- Pain
- Distress, anxiety
- Shock

Treatment
- Phone EMS.
- **Rest** – the affected body part, and reassure the victim.
- **Direct pressure** – If you are wearing gloves, apply pressure to the wound immediately using your finger or hand. If you do not have gloves, ask the victim to apply pressure to the wound. Apply a sterile dressing and bandage as soon as possible. See How to bandage, page 50.
- **Tourniquet** – When direct pressure fails to control life-threatening external limb bleeding, consider using a tourniquet.

APPLYING A TOURNIQUET:

A commercial tourniquet consists of a Velcro band and one-handed crank system to tighten the band around the circumference of the wound. Place the band just above the wound; turn the crank until bleeding stops; secure the crank into the locking position of the tourniquet. Improvise if needed by tightening a bandage (e.g. insert a pen or stick into the knot and twist) until bleeding stops.

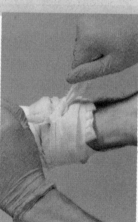

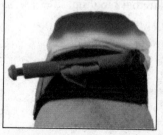

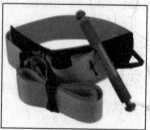

RESPIRATORY AND CIRCULATORY SYSTEMS

The anatomy and physiology of the ABCs

Airway

Airway refers to the parts of the respiratory system that connect the lungs to the "outside world." These parts include the nose, mouth, pharynx (throat), larynx (voice box or Adam's apple), and trachea (windpipe).

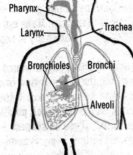

Breathing

Breathing refers to the exchange of air between the lungs and the atmosphere. The air passages consist of the nose, mouth, pharynx, larynx, trachea, bronchi, and bronchioles. These passages lead to the true lung tissues, or alveoli – the clusters of air spaces at the end of the bronchioles. In the alveoli, oxygen and carbon dioxide pass between the atmosphere and the blood. Because of the microscopic distances involved, this exchange is almost instantaneous.

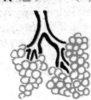

Alveoli

The lungs are elastic. When you breathe in, your lungs inflate; the diaphragm moves down, the lower rib swing outward to increa the width of the chest, and the upper ribs and breastbone move outward to increase the front-to-back diameter. Breathing out happens passively as the muscles relax.

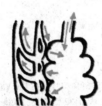

At the alveoli, oxygen and carbon dioxide are exchanged

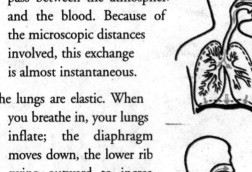

Breathing is largely automatically controlled by the "respiratory control centre," deep within the brain. The body's cells produce carbon dioxide that is picked up by the blood. The rise in blood carbon dioxide is sensed by the respiratory control centre, which causes an increase in breathing.

Circulation

The circulatory system is a closed "plumbing" system of heart, arteries, capillaries and veins through which blood flows continuously. Its purpose is to transport oxygen and other materials to the cells of the body and to remove wastes, including carbon dioxide. The circulatory system conducts blood through a simple circuit powered by two pumps working simultaneously. The pumps are the right and left ventricles of the heart.

Darker venous blood, having given up some of its oxygen to the cells, flows centrally through veins back to the heart, where it is pumped to the lungs for oxygenation. The oxygenated blood returns from the lungs to the heart and is pumped throughout the body through the aorta and arteries.

OXYGEN

Room air

21% Oxygen

Exhaled air

16% Oxygen

About 21 per cent of room air consists of oxygen. About 16 per cent of exhaled air consists of oxygen. This difference (five to six per cent) shows there is plenty of oxygen in exhaled air for use in rescue breathing to deliver to a non-breathing victim.

The circulatory system

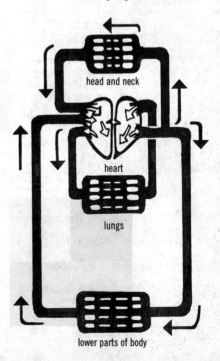

head and neck

heart

lungs

lower parts of body

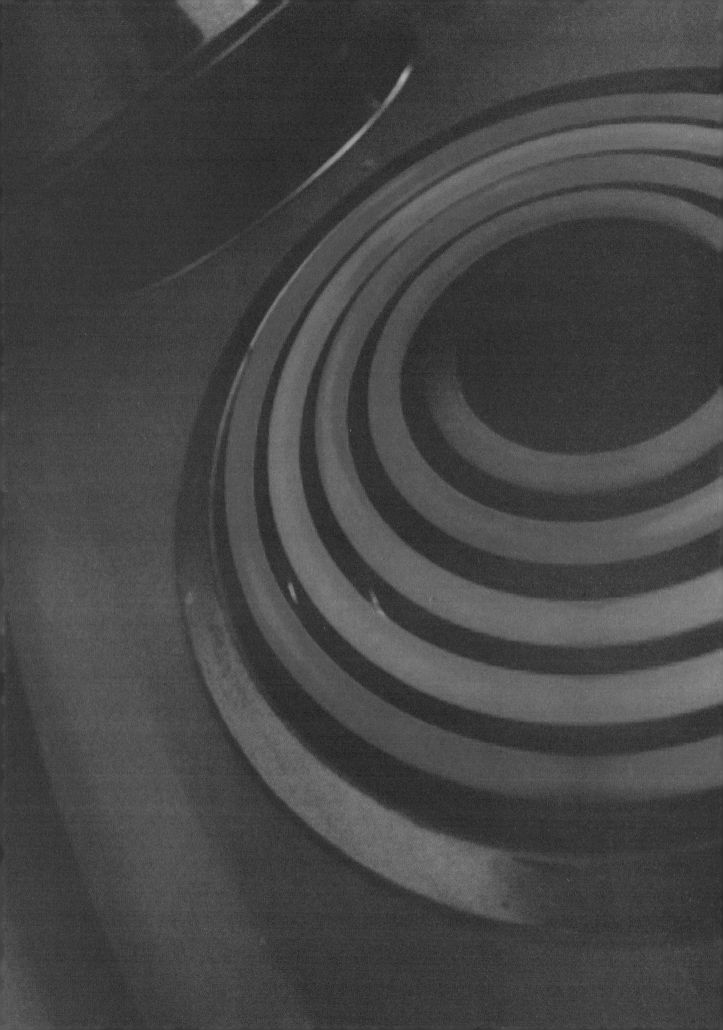

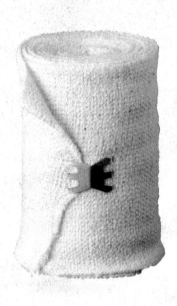

SECONDARY EMERGENCIES

RECOGNITION

ONCE ALL LIFE-THREATENING CONDITIONS HAVE BEEN ASSESSED AND TREATED, YOU CAN TEND TO OTHER CONDITIONS.

SECONDARY ASSESSMENT

SECONDARY ASSESSMENT IS A SYSTEMATIC SEARCH WITH THREE MAIN STEPS:

1. Check **vital signs**
2. Perform a **head-to-toe examination**
3. Record **relevant history – victim and incident**

The purpose of the secondary assessment is to:

- Determine what is wrong, and determine if other potential injuries, illnesses or complicating factors exist. Is the injury a result of an external force, or is this a medical disorder or illness?
- Point to the appropriate action and treatment.
- Gather information to pass on to medical or emergency personnel.

Some steps are repeated from the primary assessment. At that time, emphasis was on whether the ABCs were present or not. At the secondary assessment stage, look for more detailed information. Monitor the victim's condition, if there are changes that suggest deterioration, phone EMS and be ready to respond by performing rescue breathing or CPR.

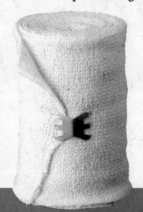

Vital signs

Vital signs provide useful clues for tracking changes in a victim's condition. Check the vital signs periodically at the beginning of the secondary assessment, then every 5–10 minutes while treating any discovered injuries. Be on alert for abnormal responses, sounds, odours, rates and rhythms, or colour and temperature shifts that may indicate a change in condition.

Check and consider these five vital signs:

1. Level of consciousness
2. Breathing 16/5sec
3. Pulse
4. Skin condition
5. Pupils

If a second rescuer or bystander is on the scene, allow that person to record vital signs and pass the results on to emergency medical personnel.

Checking the pulse

The pulse is the heartbeat. It is detectable in several places on the body where the blood vessels (especially the arteries) are close to the surface of the skin. For first aid purposes, check the victim's pulse where it is strong and where it is convenient and accessible.

These two areas are:

1. *Carotid (neck) on an adult or child:* Feel the carotid pulse in the neck next to the Adam's apple (larynx). Place two or three fingers (not your thumb) on the victim's larynx. Slide these fingers into the groove between the larynx and the muscles at the side of the neck to locate the pulse.

2. *Brachial (arm) pulse on an infant:* Feel the brachial pulse on the inside of the upper arm. Find it by gently probing the area on the inside of the arm between the muscles of the front and back of the arm (biceps and triceps).

Vital signs

How to approach Level of consciousness (LOC):

There are no strict boundaries between levels of consciousness. Simply observe, then describe how much or how well a victim responds to questions, your voice or touch. Assess i) eyes open response, ii) verbal response, and iii) motor response.

For conscious, responsive victims, ask:

Primary questions:
- Open your eyes, what is your name, can you move your fingers?

Secondary questions:
- Where are you, what time is it?
- What day is it?
- Can you tell me what happened?

For unconscious, unresponsive victims, look for:

- Do they react (open eyes, move or make a noise) when you call their name or touch them?
- Do they grasp your hand or wiggle their toes when asked?
- Do they react to painful stimuli, such as pinching?

Assess LOC:

LOC conscious and alert if the victim:
- answers coherently, is oriented to time, place and person
- eyes are open
- obeys commands

LOC conscious and confused if the victim:
- has trouble answering
- eyes open to speech or pain
- moves to pain

LOC unconscious and reacts:
- to either voice or pain
- opens eyes

LOC unconscious and does not react

Breathing

Rate	Number of breaths per minute. Normal rates are: Adults 12–20 per minute, Children 12–30, and Infants 20–30+. (Simplify by counting the number of breaths in 15 seconds and multiply by 4.)
Rhythm	Fast or slow, regular or irregular.
Depth	Deep or shallow.
Sounds	Wheezing, rasping, gurgling, any signs of pain.

Pulse

Rate	Number of beats per minute. Normal rates are: Adults 60–100 per minute, Children 80–100, Infants 100+. (Simplify by counting the number of beats in 15 seconds and multiply by 4.)
Rhythm	Regular or irregular.
Strength or quality	Strong and full, or weak and thin.

Skin

Temperature	Normal, warm-hot or cool-cold.
Moisture	Wet-clammy, profuse sweating, dry or normal.
Colour	Pale or ashen (white-grey), red-flushed or normal.

Pupils

Size	Large or small?
Equal	Are the pupils the same size?
Reactive	When exposed to light, the pupils should get smaller. Check one eye at a time by quickly covering and uncovering the eye with your hand, or by using a small flashlight.

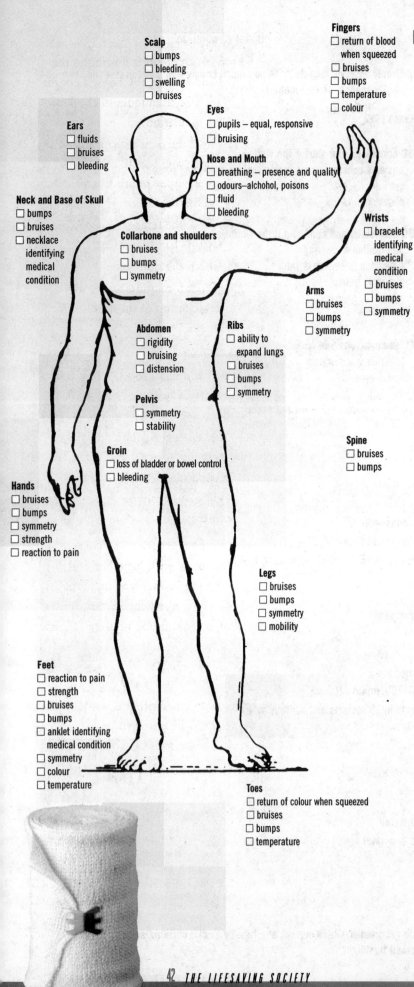

Scalp
- [ ] bumps
- [ ] bleeding
- [ ] swelling
- [ ] bruises

Ears
- [ ] fluids
- [ ] bruises
- [ ] bleeding

Eyes
- [ ] pupils – equal, responsive
- [ ] bruising

Nose and Mouth
- [ ] breathing – presence and quality
- [ ] odours–alchohol, poisons
- [ ] fluid
- [ ] bleeding

Fingers
- [ ] return of blood when squeezed
- [ ] bruises
- [ ] bumps
- [ ] temperature
- [ ] colour

Neck and Base of Skull
- [ ] bumps
- [ ] bruises
- [ ] necklace identifying medical condition

Collarbone and shoulders
- [ ] bruises
- [ ] bumps
- [ ] symmetry

Wrists
- [ ] bracelet identifying medical condition
- [ ] bruises
- [ ] bumps
- [ ] symmetry

Arms
- [ ] bruises
- [ ] bumps
- [ ] symmetry

Abdomen
- [ ] rigidity
- [ ] bruising
- [ ] distension

Ribs
- [ ] ability to expand lungs
- [ ] bruises
- [ ] bumps
- [ ] symmetry

Pelvis
- [ ] symmetry
- [ ] stability

Groin
- [ ] loss of bladder or bowel control
- [ ] bleeding

Spine
- [ ] bruises
- [ ] bumps

Hands
- [ ] bruises
- [ ] bumps
- [ ] symmetry
- [ ] strength
- [ ] reaction to pain

Legs
- [ ] bruises
- [ ] bumps
- [ ] symmetry
- [ ] mobility

Feet
- [ ] reaction to pain
- [ ] strength
- [ ] bruises
- [ ] bumps
- [ ] anklet identifying medical condition
- [ ] symmetry
- [ ] colour
- [ ] temperature

Toes
- [ ] return of colour when squeezed
- [ ] bruises
- [ ] bumps
- [ ] temperature

Head-to-toe examination

The second phase of secondary assessment is to carry out a systematic body check. Be sure to check thoroughly from head to toe because not all injuries are obvious; the position of the victim, or the nature or location of the injury may make them less apparent.

Note: *If a spinal injury is suspected, adapt your procedure to prevent movement of the head and spine.*

The examination involves touching the entire body using firm pressure to find any injury or abnormality. Although you want to be thorough with the head-to-toe check, be sensitive to a victim's anxiety and the need for privacy.

- Starting with the head, slide your hands across body surfaces with just enough pressure that you can feel below the surface.
- Use your other senses, too – touch, sight, hearing and smell.
- With responsive victims, ask permission to touch the body. If granted, constantly reassure and talk to the victim.
- Clearly indicate what you are doing. For example, "I'm just going to press down a bit on your stomach to make sure everything is OK."
- Ask questions for clarification.
- If the person does not want to be touched, use a systematic question and answer technique, and ask about all the areas of the body.
- If you have to remove clothing to expose a suspected injury, be sure to cover the area again as soon as you are finished checking.

Move the victim gently if he or she is unconscious. Talk aloud about what you are doing for recording purposes; either to tell a bystander, to tell EMS, or to help you remember when you write it down later.

Look for these signs and symptoms:

- Bumps, bruises, blood or other fluids, deformity, ability to move and temperature differences. (See the diagram on p. 42 for specific signs and symptoms to check on the body.)

- Pain, often reflected in a grimace, a wince or a verbal "ouch." Victims may hold an injury, protect it, or move away from the source of pain.

- Medical condition information (identifying conditions such as diabetes, severe allergies, heart disease).
  - Check the neck, wrists and ankles for alert medallions or bracelets.
  - Check the wallet for a card.

- Reduced or cut off circulation by checking distal circulation and sensation. "Distal" means away from the heart and refers to the circulation below the injury at the hands and feet. Impaired distal circulation is caused by certain injuries or first aid procedures. For example, a fracture may pinch an artery and restrict the flow of blood, and so may a bandage that is tied too tight. If blood is cut off from tissues below the injury, the damage could lead to loss of the limb. Check circulation before and after tying bandages and adjust as necessary.

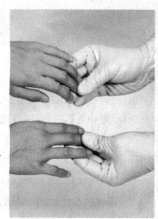

Distal circulation

How much blood is flowing to the hands and feet? Choose a couple of these techniques to check distal circulation:

- Pinch the pads or nail beds of the fingers and toes to see how quickly they return to normal pinkish colour.
- Check the temperature of the victim's hands and feet.
- Check the skin colour.
- Check for a pulse at the wrist, ankle or top of the foot.

Distal sensation

Can the victim feel a touch? To assess distal sensation:

- Squeeze, pinch or lightly brush a toe or finger – does the victim respond?
- Ask if the victim feels any tingling or numbness in the toes or fingers.

Remember to always check distal circulation and sensation in each hand and foot as part of the head-to-toe examination. Always reassess distal circulation and sensation after treating any injury to a limb.

Recording relevant history – victim and incident

This third step calls for recording the information collected during the secondary assessment. Writing down your observations helps medical personnel (or other rescuers) take over care of the victim. The history provides a reference point to assess any further changes in condition and gives an indication of the injuries.

Record as much of the following information as possible:

Incident history	Victim history
what happened and how	victim's name
any pain (location, description)	has this happened before – circumstances
injuries	medications
vital signs	allergies

S.A.M.P.L.E
Signs & Symptoms
Allergies
Medication
Past history
Last meal
Events preceding

Note: *If you are a responding to an emergency at work, you may be required to complete a first aid incident report. Ask your supervisor.*

ACTION

HELPING WITH MEDICATION

Prevent errors by checking the "5 Rights" – be sure you are using the *Right medicine*, the *Right amount* on the *Right person*, at the *Right time*, using the *Right method*.

Do NOT administer the medicine for them.

Instead:

- **get the medication for them**
- **help by opening the container**
- **physically support victims while they take the medication**

Note: Exception – a first aider may help administer an EpiPen® injector – See Severe Allergies (page 45).

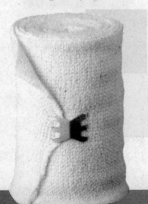

THE GOAL OF "ACTION" IS TO CARE FOR WHAT YOU FIND BY PROVIDING THE APPROPRIATE HELP OR TREATMENT.

Your initial assessment will have directed you to suspect either:

- **Illness and medical disorders** – where there is little indication of an external mishap or force, or
- **Injuries** – where it appears that an external force caused a problem.

Your secondary assessment may have identified signs and symptoms:

- **Signs** – the indications of the victim's condition that you can observe with your senses.
- **Symptoms** – the indications of the victim's condition that he or she can feel. Through a verbal assessment of the history, the victim can tell you the symptoms he or she is experiencing.

Match them to a condition and provide first aid accordingly. The following sections describe emergency conditions.

How to read the charts

All prominent signs and symptoms are listed beginning with the essentials.

The actual symptoms observed in any situation vary with the seriousness and extent of the injury or illness. Therefore, what you observe may not match everything described.

Complete the suggested treatment in the order it is written.

Other "action" steps are included along with the recommended treatment.

Remember, the information is specific to a condition and is only a part of the entire rescue process. Insert the "treatment" steps as you follow the complete step-by-step first aid process:

Check the scene and deal with ABC priorities.

Complete the secondary assessment and compare what you find with the signs and symptoms of these conditions.

Care for the secondary emergencies.

ACTION: ILLNESS AND MEDICAL DISORDERS

Severe allergies (Anaphylaxis)

Allergies become a concern for first aiders when the reaction causes sudden, severe life-threatening symptoms. The most urgent of these is the rapid onset of breathing difficulties. In these situations, victims need immediate medical attention.

Severe allergies (Anaphylaxis) – victim and incident history:

- Ask the victim specifically about allergies or check for medical condition identification.
- Suspect an allergic reaction if the victim took a new medication, ate seafood or nuts (contained in various foods), or if he or she is bitten by a bee or wasp.

Signs and symptoms

- The more signs and symptoms are present, the faster this condition develops and becomes life-threatening.
- LOC: confusion, disorientation, unconsciousness
- Breathing: difficulty, wheezing
- Tight sensation in airway
- Generalized itchiness, rash (red), hives
- Swelling of face, lips, neck or area in contact with allergen
- Nausea, vomiting
- Weakness, dizziness

Treatment

- Phone EMS.
- Ask victim if they carry an antidote kit for the allergy (e.g. auto-injector).
- Help victims with their medicine.* Asthmatics should use their auto-injector first if they suspect they are having an anaphylactic reaction.
    - Use according to the package instructions.
    - If necessary, the auto-injector will go through clothes. Massage the area to disperse the medication.
- Place used auto-injector back into the storage tube needle-first.
- Watch and monitor vital signs and changes in the victim's condition.
- A second dose may be given if signs and symptoms do not improve within 5 minutes.

AUTO-INJECTORS

An auto-injector is designed to administer a pre-measured amount of medication. Follow the manufacturer's instructions for administration.

EpiPen®

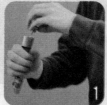 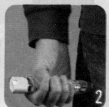

Pull off blue safety release.

Swing and firmly push orange tip again outer thigh so it clicks and hold for 10 seconds. Note the tip extends upon use covering needle.

* **Safety tip:** Protect your thumb from accidental needle puncture: cover the thumb with your fingerswhen grasping the auto-injector.

Diabetes

Diabetes is a common medical condition that affects the body's ability to regulate the level of sugar in the blood. Victims may become ill if the blood sugar level is too high or low. Diabetes is controlled through diet and insulin medication. Insulin helps carry sugar from the blood to the cells.

Diabetes – victim and incident history:
- Ask if the victim has diabetes.
- Look for medical condition identification.

Signs and symptoms	Treatment

LOC: confusion, disorientation, unconscious
Breathing: shallow, rapid
Circulation: weak, rapid pulse
Skin: sweating
Restlessness, trembling, weakness
Confusion, fear, anxiety
Nausea
Headache
May appear intoxicated
	Phone EMS.
	If unconscious, place victim in recovery position.
	If conscious, help victim test their blood sugar (if test kit is available) and help victim self-administer prescribed medication or sugar – preferably in order of:
	  Glucose tablets
	  Candy (e.g. Mentos, Skittles, Jelly beans)
	  Orange juice or other fructose juice drinks
	Advise victim to seek medical attention.
	Never administer insulin.

SEIZURES OCCURRING IN WATER

Seizures in water are potentially life-threatening because of the possibility of aspiration of water and drowning. Keep the victim's head above the surface. After the seizure, remove the victim from the water and proceed with treatment for a seizure.

Seizures

A seizure or convulsion happens when there is a large discharge of unorganized electrical impulses from the brain.

Seizures can be associated with high fevers, meningitis, stroke, brain injuries, lack of sleep, hypoglycemia (low blood sugar), diabetes, medication, drug intoxication, light (especially flickering light) and epilepsy – a disorder of the nervous system classified by seizures.

There are several types of seizures, but only the *Tonic-Clonic (Grand Mal)* variety with the symptoms listed in the chart, requires emergency first aid action. If the victim is experiencing a prolonged seizure, or repeated seizures, phone EMS.

Seizures – Tonic-Clonic (Grand Mal) – victim and incident history:
- Ask if the victim has had seizures before.
- Look for medical condition identification.

Signs and symptoms	Treatment
Tonic phase LOC: loss of consciousness Arching of the back and rigidity in the body **Clonic phase** Breathing: noisy breathing, extra saliva Contraction and relaxation of the muscles of the arms and legs (jerking or flailing) Teeth clenching or grinding Loss of control of the bowel or bladder **After seizure** Confusion, disorientation, fatigue Seldom lasts longer than three minutes	Phone EMS. Clear objects from the surrounding area to prevent the victim from striking them and getting injured. Do NOT restrict the victim's movements. Do NOT place anything between the victim's teeth. Try to record number and duration of seizures.

Fevers in infants and children

If left untreated, a high fever can cause convulsions. A convulsion is an uncontrollable abnormal muscle contraction or series of muscle contractions.

Fevers in infants and children

Signs and symptoms	Treatment
High temperature (taken in the armpit): A fever emergency occurs when a child's or infant's temperature is: ☐ 38 C (100.5 F) or higher for an infant ☐ 40 C (104 F) or higher for a child	**If the child has a fever:** ☐ Seek medical assistance or phone EMS. ☐ Advise giving acetaminophen (e.g. Tylenol®) to help reduce the child's temperature. ☐ Do not give ASA (e.g. Aspirin®) – it may cause a life-threatening condition called Reye's syndrome. ☐ Encourage the child to drink fluids. ☐ Sponge the child with lukewarm water (never cold water) for about 20 minutes – do not immerse the child or infant in a tub. ☐ Dry and dress the child in comfortable but not too warm clothes. ☐ Monitor the temperature, encourage fluids, and repeat sponging if necessary until medical help is reached or arrives. **If the child has a convulsion:** ☐ Do not restrain the child; simply protect him or her from injury by moving hard objects and guiding movements. ☐ When the convulsions stop, place the victim in the best recovery position for his or her age or size.

Unconsciousness

An unconscious victim is unresponsive to verbal or tactile stimuli and does not have the ability to clear his or her airway. A victim who has suffered any loss of consciousness should be sent to hospital.

Unconciousness

Signs and symptoms	Treatment
☐ Unresponsive to voice or pain (pinching) ☐ Unaware of surroundings	☐ Phone EMS. ☐ Identify and control cause of unconsciousness. ☐ Treat for shock. ☐ Seek medical attention.

Fainting

Fainting is a loss of consciousness due to a sudden but temporary reduction in the flow of blood to the brain.

Fainting – victim and incident history:
- Suspect a fainting spell if the victim was: in a stuffy room, standing for a long time, overly active, or stood up quickly.
- Fainting can also arise as a result of a medical disorder, stress, emotional shock or fatigue.

Signs and symptoms	Treatment
Shock: ☐ Restlessness, weakness ☐ Fear, anxiety ☐ Confusion, disorientation, unsteady ☐ Skin: pale, cold, sweaty, clammy ☐ Pulse: weak, rapid ☐ Respiration: shallow, rapid ☐ Dizziness ☐ Nausea ☐ Unconscious for less than one minute	**Before an impending faint, try to prevent injury from a fall by:** ☐ assisting the person to a lying position ☐ being ready to catch or guide them gently to the floor or ground **After fainting:** ☐ Phone EMS. ☐ Identify and control the cause of the fainting. ☐ Treat for shock. ☐ Recommend the victim seek medical attention.

BANDAGING EMBEDDED OBJECTS

With embedded objects, pressure cannot be applied directly to the wound. Pack/stack bulky dressings around the embedded object to keep it from moving while controlling bleeding. Secure the dressings in place with a narrow bandage ensuring no pressure is placed on the embedded object.

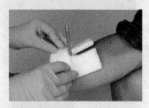

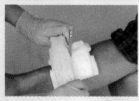

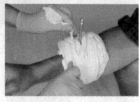

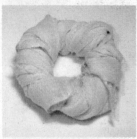

A ring pad may be useful for dealing with embedded objects. Make a narrow bandage and loop it twice around one hand. Pull the lose end through the loop, wrap it around and repeat until the entire bandage is used and you have a firm ring.

ACTION: INJURIES

Wounds

Wounds range from minor scrapes and bruises to severe cuts and internal bleeding. Minor wounds occur in every area of day-to-day life, whereas severe wounds usually occur as a result of external forces, such as an automobile crash.

Types of wounds include:

Abrasion: Scraped skin; may vary from a narrow scratch to a wide graze; bleeding is slight.

Contusion: Bruises usually caused by a hard impact from a blunt object, or a fall. Underlying tissue is damaged causing discolouration; may indicate a deeper injury.

Incision: A clean edged cut made by a sharp edge such as broken glass or knife.

Avulsion: When the wound has a flap of skin (sometimes with underlying tissue), which can be peeled back or put in place.

Laceration: A deep tearing cut with jagged edges; bleeding can be considerable. Bites from animals or humans are considered lacerations.

Puncture: A stab wound caused by sharp pointed objects penetrating the skin; may not bleed much if the embedded object acts as a plug.

Embedded objects: When objects remain in the wound (puncture or abrasion), e.g., glass, gravel, splinters, nails, knives.

Amputation: When a body part is completely, or partly, cut or torn away from the body.

External bleeding (open wound): Usually visible because blood flows through a surface wound. There are two types:

1. **Venous:** bleeding from the veins – relatively easy to stop, blood is dark red and oozes steadily.

2. **Arterial:** bleeding from the arteries – harder to control, blood is bright red and squirts.

To prevent open wounds from infection; wash your hands with soap and water, don't cough or breathe on the wound, don't touch the wound, gently clean any surface material away from the wound using slow running water, and cover the wound with a clean dressing. Signs of infection include swelling, pain, redness and pus.

Internal bleeding (closed wound): Caused by an impact or excessive pressure that does not break the skin, or from a penetrating injury (usually in the abdominal area). Because internal bleeding is not usually visible, the injury may appear slight. These injuries, however, require immediate medical attention since vital organs are injured and first aiders cannot treat the problem directly.

Wounds

Specific assessment notes: Not all wounds bleed. Head and facial wounds tend to bleed more because of the number of blood vessels.
Check for bleeding: Do an immediate visual check. Watch for blood pooling under clothes or under the body. During the secondary assessment, move your hands thoroughly under the victim (especially in hollows) and feel for damp spots.

Signs and symptoms	Treatment
Skin layer (or deeper) is broken by a scrape, cut, tear, stab, flap, bite, etc. Pain Distress, anxiety	Gently clean affected area by flushing with clean water. Apply a sterile dressing (e.g. adhesive bandage strip). For superficial wounds and abrasions apply an antibiotic ointment to promote healing unless the victim has a sensitivity to antibiotics, such as penicillin. Monitor for infection (the area around the wound becomes red, swollen or seeps pus). Consult a doctor if: 　the wound is deep or gaping (for potential stitches) 　an infection develops 　the wound is from an animal (or human) bite 　an object is stuck or embedded in the wound
Above, plus: External bleeding Shock	Control bleeding. 　**Rest** the affected body part, and reassure the victim. 　**Direct pressure** – If you are wearing gloves, apply pressure to the wound immediately using your fingers or hand. If you do not have gloves, ask the victim to apply pressure to the wound. Apply a sterile dressing and bandage as soon as possible. Check distal circulation. **Notes:** Wear gloves. Do not bandage around a neck. Maintain direct pressure with your hand. Phone EMS if there is a lot of blood loss or if you cannot control the bleeding.
Embedded objects Bleeding Pain Swelling, redness Shock	Leave the object in place. Control bleeding by applying pressure around the object – avoid pushing it in deeper. Stabilize the object to prevent further damage. Bandage the wound. Consult a doctor. For splinters and other superficial objects, remove the object with a clean instrument (e.g. a needle or tweezers) and treat the wound for bleeding or other local injury.
Amputation Jagged edges of soft tissues and bones Exposed and obviously missing body parts Complete amputation – ends of blood vessels tend to collapse resulting in surprisingly small amount of bleeding relative to the severity of the injury	If properly protected, some parts may be successfully reattached up to 24 hours after the injury. Phone EMS. Apply direct pressure to control bleeding. If direct pressure fails, use a tourniquet. Learn how to apply a tourniquet on page 36. **Partial amputation** – treat as a severe wound: reposition part to its normal position, control bleeding, cover area with moist sterile gauze, and immobilize injured part. **Complete amputation** 　If possible, recover any amputated parts. 　Wrap severed parts in moist sterile gauze and place in a sealed waterproof container. 　Place container with severed part in another container with crushed ice or ice water. 　Transport the part with the victim. 　Record time and date of the amputation.

TETANUS

If someone suffers a wound as a result of an animal bite, or you suspect a wound may be infected by contaminated soil or animal feces, advise the victim to seek medical assistance immediately. The victim may be at risk of tetanus infection – a potentially fatal disease characterized by muscle spasms.

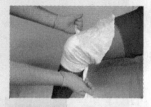

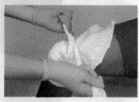

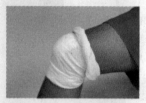

Knee or elbow bandage

Hold the dressing in place with a triangular bandage: lay the triangular bandage on the dressing with the point of the triangle on the thigh; wrap the two bandage ends under the knee and tie them together on top of the point above the knee.

Pull the point up the thigh to apply pressure to the dressing and tuck the point over and under the knotted bandage ends, or alternately secure the point to the knot with a safety pin.

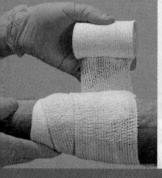

A roller bandage is gauze-like material used to secure a dressing.

Internal bleeding – victim and incident history

Check for internal bleeding whenever the victim has experienced a heavy, hard impact, or been struck by a solid physical blow. While we may expect internal bleeding as part of multiple injuries, do not rule it out as a single grievance if no other injury seems present.

Signs and symptoms	Treatment
☐ Breathing: short of breath	☐ Phone EMS.
☐ Skin: sweating, discolouration or bruising	☐ Treat for shock.
☐ LOC: decreased level of consciousness	
☐ Abdominal muscle spasm or rigid abdomen	
☐ Swelling	
☐ Pain in the abdomen or injury site	
☐ Shock	
☐ Anxiety	

Bandaging

Use a sterile dressing to soak up the blood and then tie it using a bandage to maintain direct pressure. Keep the dressing in place.

Dressings

- Many first aid kits stock dressings. They are usually made of gauze and individually packaged to keep them sterile. Various sizes are available. Kerchiefs, scarves, gloves and T-shirts also work. Look for the cleanest material available. Other desirable characteristics are: absorbent, lint free, larger than the wound, thick and soft enough to evenly distribute pressure.

Bandages

- Common commercial bandages include: elastic tensor bandage, gauze roll, adhesive tape and a triangular bandage folded into a long strip. Ties, scarves and anything you improvise will also work in a pinch.

How to bandage

- Cover the entire dressing so pressure is distributed evenly.
- Make a **triangular bandage** by cutting a piece of square material (approximately one-metre square) in half to produce two triangles. Fold the point to the centre of the base, allowing the point to extend just beyond the base, and fold again from the top to make a **broad bandage**. Fold a broad bandage in half again from the top to the base to make a **narrow bandage**.
- Wrap the bandage around the victim to secure it. Tie the ends of the bandage in a knot on top of the dressing and the wound.
- **Tie it securely, but not so tight that it blocks distal circulation.** Loosen the bandage if the parts beyond the bleeding area are getting cool, turning pale, or lack a pulse.
- Do not lift the bandage; this may disturb any clots that are starting to develop. If blood starts to seep through all the material, add another bandage on top.

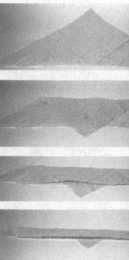

Slings

A sling is a good idea if the victim is going to be transported by someone other than EMS, such as rescuer or family member. If EMS personnel are transporting the victim, let them support and immobilize any injuries.

The simplest form of sling is a belt or broad scarf looped around the wrist and neck. For better support and comfort, use a triangular cloth (triangular bandage or square scarf folded into a triangle) or commercial arm sling.

Slings for shoulder, collarbone or hand injuries

1. On the injured side, bend the victim's elbow so the hand rests on top of the breastbone in the middle of the chest.
2. Facing the victim, hold the middle and top edge of the sling. Position it over the arm pointing to the injured side over the elbow, with the straight edge hanging vertically along the opposite side.
3. Pull the bottom point gently under the injured arm to form a "tube" to support the forearm. Secure under the fingers and elbow.
4. Pull it over the injured-side shoulder and tie at the hollow of the neck.
5. The weight should be on the elbow.

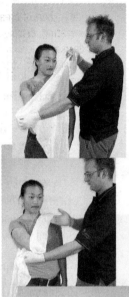
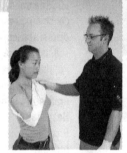
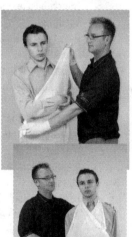

Slings for lower arm or wrist

1. Bend the elbow so the forearm is horizontal.
2. Facing the victim, hold the middle and top edge of the sling. Position it between the arm and body with the pointing side under the elbow, with the straight edge hanging vertically along the opposite side.
3. Pull the lower point up and over the arm, past the shoulder and behind the neck.
4. Adjust the arm to a comfortable angle and tie the two points at the hollow of the neck.
5. If possible, leave the fingers visible.

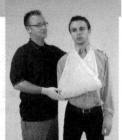
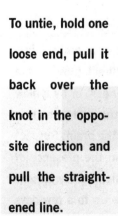

To provide comfort and reduce movement, pad hollow spaces and pad underneath the tied knot on the shoulder. For padding, use a folded cloth, towels, mittens or readily available material. Place the padding under the elbow or wherever there are gaps between the sling and the body.

TYING A REEF KNOT

Reef knots are best for tying bandages and slings because they lie flat (for comfort), don't slip, and are easy to untie.

- Hold one end of the bandage in each hand.
- Pass the left end over the right end and tuck it under.
- Then pass the same end, now in the right hand, over the left end and tuck it under.

Remember: Left over Right and under, then Right over Left and under. You may also start from the right, i.e. Right over Left and under, then Left over Right and under.

To untie, hold one loose end, pull it back over the knot in the opposite direction and pull the straightened line.

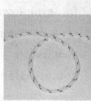

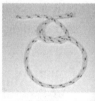
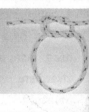

BUMPS ON THE HEAD

These injuries are common, especially among children, and should be taken seriously in case there is underlying damage to the skull or brain. Usually the injury is harmless and any discolouration and swelling disappears within hours. But if you suspect the impact was hard enough to cause serious damage, treat it as a head injury. Watch for symptoms of a fracture, concussion or compression. Seek medical attention if in doubt, otherwise, use a cold compress or ice bag to relieve pain and swelling.

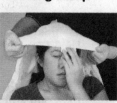
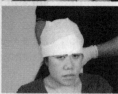
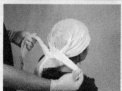
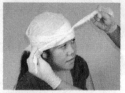
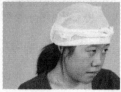

CONCUSSION

A concussion is a brain injury caused by a direct blow to the head, face, or neck, or by a blow elsewhere on the body which is transmitted to the brain. Suspect a concussion in the presence of one or more signs or symptoms which can take up to a few days to appear.

Head injuries

Head injuries are caused in three general ways:
1. The victim's head hits an object (e.g. from falling or diving).
2. An object hits the head (e.g. a hockey puck, baseball bat or candlestick).
3. Vigorous shaking.

The injury may be of two types, which may occur separately or together:
1. Surface injuries affecting skin and bones.
2. Brain injury such as bleeding within the brain or just under the skull (compression injury); or a blow transmitted to the head (concussion injury).

Head injuries – victim and incident history:
- The more serious the head injury, the more likely there will be neck and spinal injuries as well. Treat for the most serious of combinations.
- A seemingly minor head injury can lead to serious complications if there is lengthy delay without treatment. Watch for the severity of the symptoms to increase.
- A serious injury may occur without any obvious visible signs. Pay close attention to incident history and level of consciousness.

Signs and symptoms

- LOC: decreased level of consciousness, confusion, disorientation, loss of consciousness, seizure
- Pupils: unequal in size or do not get smaller when exposed to light
- Head pain
- Bleeding, swelling, or bruising
- Blurred vision, nausea and vomiting
- Anxiety, agitation
- Shock
- Blood or clear fluid from the eyes, ears, nose or mouth

Concussion (temporary disturbance of brain function) – above, plus:
- Victim claims to "see stars"
- Loss of memory of events around the time of injury

Compression (pressure on the brain caused by a buildup of fluids or a depressed skull fracture) – above, plus:
- Symptoms are progressive and usually get worse over time

Treatment

- Phone EMS.
- Immobilize spine if you suspect a neck or spinal injury (see Spinal injuries).
- Treat the area for bleeding, bruising or swelling. If you suspect a skull fracture, do not apply direct pressure – simply apply a thick dressing.
- For a suspected concussion, stop the sport or recreational activity and seek medical help.

While waiting for EMS:
- Continue to check level of consciousness (What's your name? What happened? Where are you?), pulse and respiration.
- Check for painful areas, loss of feeling, tingling, as well as response to sound, touch and other stimuli.
- If bleeding from nose, mouth or ears, protect the airway
- If a skull fracture is suspected, control bleeding with a thick dressing, but do not apply direct pressure.

Head bandages – How to:
- Place a dressing on the scalp wound.
- Using a triangular bandage, stand behind the victim and place the base of the bandage in the middle of the victim's forehead, close to the eyebrows.
- Bring the point side of the bandage over the head to cover the dressing.
- Bring the ends around the back of the head, cross them over the point and back around the head to the front. Tie the two ends using a reef knot low on the forehead.
- Keep the victim's head steady with your hand and pull the point down to adjust the amount of pressure on the dressing.
- Fold the point up and secure it to the top part of the bandage with a safety pin, or tuck it under the crossed part of the bandage at the back.

Spinal injuries

Spinal injuries affect the backbone. They can include any neck, upper or lower back injury. Common causes of spinal injuries include:

- Severe head injuries.
- Falls – including falling backwards, landing in a sitting position, or while intoxicated.
- Crashes (e.g. in a car, on a bicycle, playing sports).
- Diving head-first into shallow water – hitting the bottom or some other object such as a rock, sandbar or large garbage item.
- Other water activity – being thrown in.

The possibility of a spinal injury complicates first aid efforts. It is necessary to protect the spinal column from further injury to avoid potential damages, particularly paralysis.

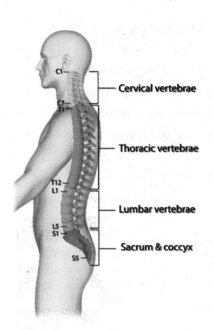

Cervical vertebrae

Thoracic vertebrae

Lumbar vertebrae

Sacrum & coccyx

Spinal injuries

Scene assessment

- Assess potential spinal injuries at the very beginning when approaching an emergency scene to ensure the victim is moved as little as possible during primary and secondary assessments.
- Victim and incident history.
- If in doubt, treat as a spinal injury.
- Do not hesitate to suspect a spinal injury even if the victim is conscious, or walking or moving after a fall, or hitting their head.

Signs and symptoms	Treatment
Pain at the site of the injury	Phone EMS.
Pain, with or without movement	Immobilize in position found – do not move the victim unless there is no other choice, i.e., to move to safety, to open the airway or to perform CPR.
Loss of coordination or movement in parts beyond the injury	Ask victim to remain still.
Weakness or altered sensation such as numbness or tingling – affecting one or both sides of the body	ABCs for suspected spinal injuries – open airway with head-tilt/chin-lift.
Bruising, swelling, or bleeding at the site of the injury	Stabilization.
Lying on the back with arms stretched above the head	Transport to hospital.
Abnormal positioning, twisted, deformity	
Abnormal muscle actions or joint stability	
Impaired breathing	
Involuntary loss of bowel and bladder control	
Shock	

If the victim is in the water	The principles above apply. For specific techniques, refer to *Aquatic spinal injury management* later in this section.

If the victim vomits	Clear the airway by turning the victim; avoid twisting or moving the neck and spine.
	Recruit assistance to hold the head, neck, and back in line.
	Turn victim to the side as a single unit.
	Use a finger sweep to clear the airway.

Treatment details for spinal injuries

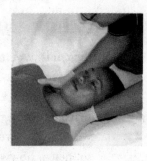

Immobilization: If at all possible, immobilize a spinal injury victim in the position found until EMS arrives.

Some circumstances will require moving the victim. This is usually a "life over limb" situation where the only way to save a victim is to move him or her. For example:

- when environmental hazards pose risk of further injury to the victim or rescuer
- when CPR is required

Maintaining immobilization: The victim needs to be still during all treatment and assessments. Here are some tips:

- **Talk to the victim** – ask the victim to be still and not move. Be reassuring. Help the victim understand what is happening by describing what you are doing.
- **Hold** – assign a bystander to gently, but firmly, hold the victim's head still and maintain head-neck-back alignment.
- **Pack** – support, prop and secure the victim in place with blankets, clothing, walls, chairs, etc.
- **Pad** – support and pad each side of the body and any injured or hollow areas using sandbags, books, rolled up blankets, towels or clothing.

ABCs – modifications for suspected spinal injured victims: Checking for breathing does not always require rolling the victim onto his or her back. A cry of pain, chest movement, or the sound of breathing tells you the victim is breathing.

- **Airway** – try to maintain an airway without extending the neck.
  - **Breathing** – if the victim is breathing, monitor closely. If the victim is not breathing, open airway with head-tilt/chin-lift. Alternatively, jaw thrust may be used by rescuers who are trained in this technique (see page 24).

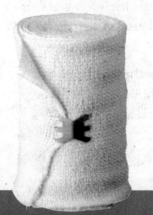

Spineboard stabilization: Stabilization refers to the victim being placed face-up on a firm surface such as a spineboard. This maintains immobilization during transportation to hospital. Ideally, allow EMS personnel to stabilize the victim. First aiders should stabilize a victim on a spineboard only if it is required to move the victim out of a life-threatening situation.

Objective

- The goal is to transfer the victim without twisting or moving the spine.

Requirements

- 3–5 people
- Spineboard, or improvise with a door or similar flat, hard "stretcher."
- Straps: luggage straps, belts, scarves, etc.

Readying the spineboard

- Lay the board beside the victim.
- Put straps underneath the board, ready to wrap around the board and victim.

Positioning rescuers

- Position a rescuer on the side of the board opposite the victim, ready to move it under the victim.
- Put one rescuer at the head of the victim – kneel at the top of the head, grip the victim's shoulders with the head resting between your forearms, and squeeze firmly like a vice.
- Position others in line on the same side of the victim – place them first at the shoulders and hips. Place extra people at the knees, back and feet.

Log-roll method

- Decide on a signal, such as "one, two, three, roll." Designate a leader to call out the signal. On the signal (e.g. "roll"), rescuers roll the victim towards them so the victim is on his or her side. Consider the weight of each part of the body and follow the speed of the person at the hips. The rescuer at the head twists along with the victim, maintaining the hold, keeping the victim's head in line with the backbone.

- The rescuer with the board slides it gently across so that it meets the victim.
- The leader signals again, "one, two, three, roll." Rescuers gently roll the victim back down, this time, on the board.

Immobilize and move

- Strap across the chest first, then strap the hips and legs.
- Stabilize the head and neck by packing in place with rolled up blankets, towels or clothing.
- Strap the forehead and packing to the board.
- Arrange rescuers on both sides of the victim, starting from the shoulders and hips.
- Put extra people at the legs and feet.
- Lift the board together (use a signal and designate a leader).
- Rescuers should bend their knees and lift using their leg muscles to protect their backs.
- Keep the victim as level as possible.
- To protect fingers when putting the board and victim down, lower the spineboard to about 5 cm above the ground or platform. Let the person at the head put the board down first, then people on the sides, then at the feet.

Aquatic spinal injury management

As a first aider, you may find yourself at the scene of a water-related emergency, perhaps in a backyard pool, at the beach or in a boat. You may be first on the scene or in a situation where a lifeguard(s) needs your assistance. If so, here is how you can assist in first aid for aquatic-related spinal injuries.

Spinal injuries complicate first aid efforts on land. Spinal injuries in the water add additional complexity because rescuers must keep the victim's head above water while contending with immobilization.

Spinal injuries can result in paralysis or death. Fortunately, injuries to the head and spine are infrequent, though they are predictable. Diving into shallow water is one of the leading causes of spinal injuries – the force of hitting the bottom usually breaks the neck. The diver may not know the water is shallow, may hit a sandbar or something hidden on the bottom, or may simply perform a poor dive.

Prevention

- Know the area – know the depth. Is it over your head? Is anything in the way? Are there submerged hazards like rocks, a cement block, an old pier support or garbage? If you don't know, don't dive.
- Check the water every time you dive because water levels change, tides flow, sandbars move, garbage comes and goes. In a crowded swimming area, check that the entire path of your dive is clear of toys and people.
- Keep your arms over your head for the entire path of your dive.
- Just learning? Always practice in water well over your head. This provides extra space if the dive goes off course.
- Expert diver? Nevertheless, make it a rule to dive into deep water only. Besides skill, slippery surfaces, fatigue, heat, cold and illness can affect your performance.
- In a lifeguarded setting, follow the rules.

Aquatic assessment – victim and incident history

Is there a spinal injury? Look for clues at the emergency scene. If the answer to any of the following questions is "yes," suspect a spinal injury and treat it as such.

Where is the victim?

- where the waves break at a beach or wave pool
- in shallow water (pool, hot tub, lake, ocean, dugout, backyard pool)
- within 3–4 metres from any edge (e.g. pool edge, raised shoreline, dock)
- at the bottom of a slide, under a diving board, below a swing or Tarzan rope
- collision in a water slide, collisions with other swimmers
- in line with a starting block (used for competitive races)
- on pool steps or a ramp entrance
- under or beside a raft, inflatable toy, or anything you can climb onto and dive or fall from

How is the victim positioned?

- limp, little or no movement
- floating under water or just below the surface
- face-up or hanging face-down like a rag doll

What happened? Can the victim or bystanders tell you about the injury?

- did the victim dive in?
- did the victim enter the water from a height?
- did the victim tumble in head first?

Treatment for aquatic spinal injuries

Proper treatment of a victim with spinal injuries requires the coordination of many skills in a sequence that:

- immobilizes the spine
- maintains the airway, breathing, and circulation
- allows for removal and transportation to hospital or other medical facility

Use judgment in deciding how and when to stabilize a victim using a rollover, and when to use a spineboard. Factors to consider when making these decisions include the number of rescuers available, the victim's condition, and the water and weather conditions.

Aquatic spinal injuries

Signs and symptoms	Treatment sequence (full details follow)
Breathing: impaired breathing	Phone EMS – send bystander.
Loss of coordination or movement in parts beyond the injury	Approach.
Pain at the site of the injury	Immobilization and rollover (if necessary).
Weakness, numbness or tingling	ABCs – airway, breathing, and circulation.
Abnormal positioning	Stabilization.
Abnormal muscle actions or joint stability	Removal.
Loss of bowel and bladder control	Treatment for shock.
Shock	Further treatment.

While the ABCs are listed fourth in the sequence, they are still the priority. This means you must do the first three steps efficiently so the ABC priorities can be assessed, treated and monitored.

1. **Contact EMS:** Send a second rescuer or bystander to contact EMS.

2. **Approach:** Slip into the water. Approach the victim carefully to minimize water movement. Do not jump or dive into the water near the victim.

3. **Immobilization and rollover:** When the victim is on his or her back, or floating with the face up, a rollover is unnecessary. If the victim is face down or partially submerged, you may need to roll him or her over to

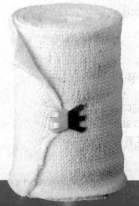

assess and maintain the ABCs and to immobilize the head and neck. The objective is to align or realign the head and spine in a straight line.

Techniques for immobilization and rollovers

While there are a variety of aquatic immobilization and rollover techniques, these two are suitable for a lone rescuer and make assessing breathing easier. Choose one of these two: i) *Canadian rollover and immobilization technique, or ii) Vice grip immobilization and rollover technique.* Modify the basic technique depending on the number of rescuers and maintain your objectives to:

- reduce or prevent movement of the victim's head and neck

- allow you to assess and monitor the ABCs
- allow you to do rescue breathing
- allow you to hold the victim's body at, or just below the surface

Basic techniques do NOT work if:

- you feel resistance when trying to move the head
- the victim complains of pain-like pressure or muscle spasms when you first try to move the head
- the victim's head is severely angled

In these cases, do NOT move the victim's head in line with the body, instead, support the victim's head in the position you found it.

Canadian rollover and immobilization technique

Number of rescuers needed: one, two or three.

Advantages: Useful when the victim is in very shallow water and the victim is much smaller than the rescuer, for example, an adult rescuer and a child victim.

Limitations: May not be suitable for victims with bulky or muscular shoulders because the extended arms may not be able to squeeze the victim's head.

Concept: The victim's head and neck are splinted between the victim's arms, extended beyond the head.

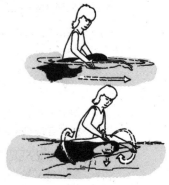

How to:

- Stand beside the victim.
- Grasp the victim's arms midway between the elbow and the shoulder — your right hand on the victim's right arm, your left hand on the victim's left arm.
- Gently float the victim's arms up alongside his or her head, parallel to the water surface.
- Position the victim's arms so they extend against his or her head.
- Squeeze and hold the arms tightly against the victim's head.
- Gently roll the victim toward you until he or she is face up.
- Brace the victim's head in the crook of your arm.
- Assess the victim's breathing.

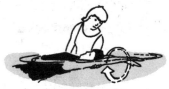

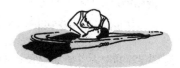

Vice grip immobilization and rollover technique

Number of rescuers needed: one, two or three.

Limitations: When there is only one rescuer who is much smaller than the victim, it may be difficult or even impossible to assess the ABCs and perform rescue breathing.

Concept: The victim is sandwiched front to back between the rescuer's forearms.

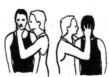 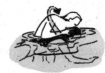 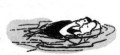

How to:

- Stand beside the victim, and face his or her head.
- Lower your body, until your shoulders are at water level.
- Reach into the water with one arm and place your forearm along his or her breastbone. Place your other forearm along the spine.
- The hand in front supports the chin: the thumb is on one side, the fingers on the other.
- At the same time, use the other hand to support the victim's head at the back of the skull. To do this, spread the fingers and cradle the head.
- Lock both your wrists, squeeze your forearms together, and clamp the victim's chest and back between your forearms and hands.
- Turn the victim face up by keeping your hands in position and rotating the victim toward you while you start to lower yourself in the water.
- Carefully roll under the victim while turning him or her over in the water. The victim is face up when stabilized.

ABC priorities

Because you need to minimize movement when dealing with victims with suspected spinal injuries, here are some notes and technical modifications to use for rescue breathing.

ABCs are the priority, so if the only way you can perform rescue breathing or CPR is by moving the neck and spine, do so. It is a matter of "life over limb," i.e., saving the life comes before saving the limb or treating a non-life-threatening injury.

Airway

- Make sure the airway is clear of foreign objects.
- If the victim is not breathing, open the airway using the head-tilt/chin-lift or jaw thrust if trained.
- Be prepared for the victim to vomit. (Vomiting is a common complication involving drowning and spinal injury.) If you are in the water, protect the airway from water entering. Roll the victim to the side as one unit, either in your hold or on a spineboard. If other rescuers are present, they should help by supporting the body. This can be done either in your hold or on a spineboard. Do a finger sweep of the mouth.

Breathing

If you can tell that a person is breathing – either because you hear the breath, see some movement around the chest, or the victim talks, blinks or murmurs with pain – do not move him or her.

If you have a victim immobilized in a spinal hold, monitor breathing closely. Injuries to the neck could affect breathing.

- If the victim is not breathing, or if you are unsure about it, open the airway. Check for breathing and begin rescue breathing if necessary.
- When to start? Begin in shallow water as soon as possible.

Circulation

If, after giving two breaths, the victim remains unresponsive and non-breathing, start CPR (chest compressions and breaths).

- Remove the victim from the water immediately to initiate CPR. A spineboard removal is not required when CPR is indicated.

Stabilization on a spineboard

With several rescuers available, use a spineboard (if available) to remove a breathing victim from the water.

While in the water, transfer the victim from your hold to a spineboard. Strap the victim securely to the board. In the absence of a spineboard, wait for EMS if possible. If you expect EMS will take too long, look for materials you can use to "splint" from head to chest, to hips to toes.

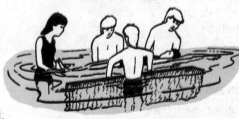

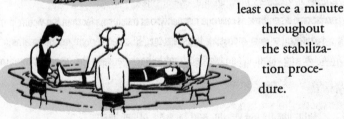

Two or three rescuers are needed for effective stabilization. A sample technique for stabilization follows. Procedures will vary depending on factors such as the victim's condition, rescuer's skill, the number of rescuers and the equipment available. It is important to remember to check the ABCs at least once a minute throughout the stabilization procedure.

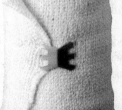

Sample stabilization technique

- Rescuer 1 has the victim immobilized and is checking and rechecking breathing.
- Rescuer 2 moves to hold the victim's hips and thighs up.
- Rescuer 3 holds the victim's feet up.
- Rescuer 4 brings the spineboard into the water and approaches the victim from the side.
- Rescuer 4 holds the board under the water so that it doesn't bump the victim. He or she then slides the board under the victim and positions it lengthwise along the victim's spine. The board is allowed to rise under the victim.
- Rescuer 3 places a hand on each side of the victim's head to help minimize movement as Rescuer 1 slowly and carefully withdraws his or her hands from the victim's head.
- Rescuers 1 and 4 secure chest straps snugly under the victim's armpits.
- Hip straps are secured with the victim's arms at his or her sides. The victim's head is secured on both sides. If the board has a head harness, it is used. Sandbags, rolled towels, etc., may also be used. Do not move the head while it is being secured.
- All remaining straps are secured at the thighs and feet.

USE OF SPINEBOARDS

Spineboards, also known as backboards, are often used as a removal device for a victim with a suspected spinal injury. EMS will use additional assessment protocols and may remove the spineboard when preparing to transport the victim.

Removal

Whenever possible, a person with a suspected spinal injury should be removed from shallow water. Removal requires at least two rescuers if a spineboard is involved, although having three or four rescuers is preferred.

Any removal procedure that allows for efficient, careful removal is appropriate. "Careful" removal implies safety to the rescuers, too. Rescuers need to use safe lifting techniques; lift using leg muscles and keep fingers from crunching between the spineboard and the ground or floor. Start in the water with these basic steps:

- If possible, recruit bystanders to help. Position them on land.
- Position the board head first, at right angles to the pool or dock edge.
- The board is removed head first, as horizontal as possible throughout.
- The rescuer at the victim's head should direct the removal by instructing all other rescuers to:
  - position themselves so the greatest lifting power is beside the victim's head and chest
  - check that their grip is secure
  - lift at an agreed upon signal (e.g. "on the count of 3")
  - lift up and gently move the victim and board out of the water
- Be prepared for the victim to vomit as a result of removal. To drain the mouth, roll the board and victim as one unit. Sweep the mouth with a hooked finger.

Treat for shock

Because a serious head or spinal injury can affect the body's heating and cooling mechanisms, victims with spinal injuries are susceptible to shock. Offer reassurance, let them rest, and provide warmth by patting them dry and covering with dry towels or blankets.

Further action

Do a secondary assessment. Treat any other injuries.

Facial injuries

Injuries to the facial area, including the mouth, nose, ears and eyes, require specialized treatment to protect the victim's vital sense organs. These injuries include:

- Dental and mouth
- Ear
- Nosebleeds and nose
- Eye

Facial injuries – general

Signs and symptoms	Treatment
Breathing: airway may be blocked by blood, vomit or dentures	Get medical assistance.
Scrape, cut, tear, stab, flap, bite, crushed	If a neck injury is suspected, immobilize and ensure open airway.
Pain	If victim is unconscious or has severe facial injury, assume there is a neck injury as well, and care for as a spinal injury.
Distress, anxiety	Control bleeding with gentle direct pressure in case bones are broken.
Bleeding	

Dental and mouth injury

Signs and symptoms	Treatment
Breathing: airway may be blocked by teeth fragments	Ensure airway is open:
Broken or missing teeth	Look for any obstructions in the mouth.
Cut tongue	Check if the tongue is bleeding.
	Keep blood and saliva drained away from the throat by tilting the head forward or placing the victim in the recovery position.
	Teeth can be salvaged. Hold tooth from the crown. Do not clean to avoid damaging the roots. Place in a balanced salt solution (e.g. Hank's Salt Solution). Alternatives include egg white, coconut water, whole milk, or saline. Otherwise, store tooth in victim's own saliva (not in the mouth). Do not reinsert the tooth: it can injure the victim or harm the tooth.
	Advise victim to see a dentist for medical follow-up.

If you cannot seal the victim's mouth to perform rescue breathing, modify your technique:
- Mouth-to-nose: close the victim's mouth and seal your mouth around the victim's nose.
- Other rescue breathing steps remain the same.

Ear injuries

Signs and symptoms	Treatment
Foreign object in ear	Remove object gently only if it can be easily seen and grasped.
	Avoid flushing an object from an ear as it could swell and cause more damage (e.g. beans or seeds).
	Adjust victim to allow drainage.
	If the object remains stuck, do not remove it yourself. Get medical assistance.
	Control bleeding of external wounds (use direct pressure).
Cuts or tears	Cover with sterile cloth and bandage.
Bleeding	If the bleeding is internal, adjust the dressing to allow drainage. This will avoid pressure from developing inside the ear.
Bruises	Advise victim to see a doctor.
	If all or part of the ear is amputated, place the ear tissue in a dry plastic bag, put it in ice water and call EMS.

Nosebleeds and nose injuries

Nosebleeds are generally caused by a hit to the nose, or they can start spontaneously.

Signs and symptoms	Treatment
Blood from the nose Pain associated with being hit Anxiety Shock	Pinch nose firmly with thumb and forefinger just above the nostrils (where the nasal bone and cartilage meet), head tilted slightly forward. Hold (or get victim to hold) firmly for at least 20 minutes to allow a clot to form. Phone EMS if the nosebleed lasts more than 20 minutes or if the victim is distressed.
Foreign object in nose	Remove object gently only if it can be easily seen and grasped. Advise victim to get medical assistance if object is far up the nose. Do NOT try to remove it.

Eye injuries

Immediate and proper first aid may prevent partial or complete loss of eyesight. Always take special care around eye injuries because the area is very sensitive.

Eye injuries often result from dust, an eyelash or other small particle lodging on the surface of the eyeball. To prevent eye injuries, wear safety glasses when you work with tools or when you play sports, and keep dangerous chemicals off high shelves.

Signs and symptoms	Treatment
General Pain in or around the eye Swelling, redness, bleeding, or other injury Eye feels scratchy or burning Increased movement of eye Uncontrollable tearing Sensitive to light, impaired vision Anxiety	Phone EMS if there is an object in the eye or vision is affected. If the eye area is wounded, treat the injury. Wash your hands. Do not remove contact lenses. Just make a note for EMS.

Floating foreign object in eye

Eyelid
Pupil
Sclera
Iris

Ciliary Muscle
Cornea
Iris
Lens
Aqueous Humour
Sclera
Medial Rectus Muscle
Lateral Rectus Muscle
Retina
Choroid
Macula
Optic Nerve
Vitreous Humour

Do not remove a foreign object manually or take any action that might embed an object deeper.
If a foreign object is floating in the eye, try flushing the eye with clean, skin temperature water.
To remove a particle from the **upper eyelid**, tell the victim to pull the upper lid over the lower lid, then let go. This may sweep the particle out. If not, use a cotton-tipped applicator at the base of the upper lid and carefully press backwards. Hold the upper eyelashes and pull the lid back over the applicator to expose the underside of the eyelid. If you can see the particle, remove it with a moist tissue, cloth or applicator.
To remove a particle from the **lower eyelid**, pull the lower eyelid down away from the eyeball while the victim rolls the eye upward. If you can see the particle, remove it with a moist tissue, cloth or applicator.
To remove a particle from the **eyeball**, shine a light across the eye (not into it) and look for the particle. If the particle is loose and not on the centre of the eye, remove it with a moist tissue, cloth or applicator.

In every case, if you've removed something from a victim's eye and the pain continues, get medical help.

Bandage* the affected eye.
Encourage the victim to keep his or her eyes still, i.e., look around with the head, not the eyes.
Keep the victim from rubbing the eye(s).
Advise victim to seek medical attention.

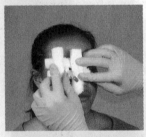
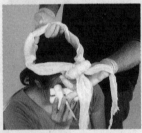
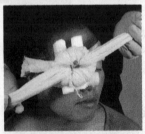
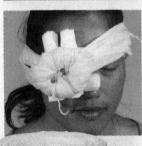
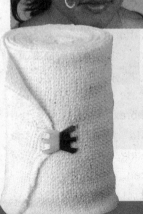

* About bandaging eyes
The goal is to prevent further injury by reducing eye movement, yet still providing reassurance. Bandage an eye by placing a shield or protective cup over it. (The bandage should not apply pressure to the eye.) Secure the patch with tape or a bandage, which is wrapped around the head, avoiding the neck. Tie it at the back of the head, not over the eye.

Eye injuries, continued

Signs and symptoms	Treatment
Chemicals spilled in the eye	◻ Phone EMS. ◻ Flush the eye(s) with skin temperature running water for 15–20 minutes – continue during transport to hospital.
Object embedded in eyeball	◻ Phone EMS. ◻ Do not try to remove object. ◻ Do not apply any pressure to the eye or eyelids. ◻ Bandage* both eyes if the victim agrees, bandage affected eye if victim objects to having both eyes covered. If an object is protruding beyond the bones surrounding the eye, "extend" that protective socket before bandaging. Use the bottom of a paper cup or place padding around the eye following the eyebrow and cheekbones. If you don't have a paper cup, use a ring pad (see p. 48) and triangular bandage to hold the dressing in place. ◻ Encourage the victim to keep his or her eyes still, i.e., look around with the head, not the eyes.
Extruded eyeball	◻ Phone EMS. ◻ If the eyeball is out of its socket, do not attempt to put it back in. ◻ Cover the eyeball with a moist dressing. Hold it in place with tape, more dressings, a cup or a ring pad bandage. ◻ Immobilize the victim's head and move him or her by stretcher (face up). ◻ Keep the victim calm.

Chest and abdominal injuries

Our rib cage protects our organs, so the ribs often fail first if we are struck in the chest. More powerful impacts may affect internal organs. Types of chest or abdominal injuries include:

- **Open chest wound** – when the chest wall is punctured leaving a hole in the chest cavity. Breathing efforts may suck air in and out of the chest through the wound.
- **Collapsed lung** – from a fall or blow with a blunt object. Air is in the chest cavity, but outside the lung.
- **Broken ribs** – from a direct impact or some kind of crushing action.
- **Abdominal injuries** – from a forceful blow, blast or severe fall that does not break the skin. Instead, the organs or tissues are wounded and bleed internally. This bleeding stays inside the abdominal cavity unseen, causing further injury and shock. There may be little or no sign of external injury.
- **Genital Injuries** – any wound or injury in this area is especially sensitive, both physically and emotionally. First aiders should be sensitive to victim reactions when treating these injuries.

Chest and abdominal injuries
For specific injuries, insert the specific treatment into the step-by-step rescue process.

Signs and symptoms	Treatment
Common to all chest injuries ☐ Breathing: difficult, short of breath ☐ Swelling, bruising or bleeding ☐ Pain at the site of the injury ☐ Shock	☐ Phone EMS. ☐ Help the victim into the most comfortable position. ☐ Protect and support the injured area. ☐ Be sensitive to the victim's privacy. ☐ Monitor for changes. Be prepared to perform rescue breathing if breathing stops. ☐ Do not give any food or liquids.
Open chest wound ☐ A puncture-type injury (e.g. fall on a sharp object, gunshot, etc.) ☐ An open wound ☐ A sucking sound when the victim breathes in ☐ Blood or blood-stained bubbles at the wound when the victim breathes out	Perform common treatment for chest injuries, above. *Specifics:* ☐ Only apply a non-occlusive* dressing. Change dressing immediately if it becomes blood-soaked. Alternatively, leave the wound exposed to prevent a tension pneumothorax (see sidebar). Apply direct pressure only if there is massive external bleeding. * A non-occlusive dressing is non-adhering and permeable allowing liquids or gasses to pass through.
Broken ribs ☐ Breathing: rapid, shallow ☐ Pain at point of injury or a springy feeling to the rib cage when gently pressed ☐ Moving, coughing or deep breathing causes pain ☐ Victim wants to stay still and tends to favour the injured area ☐ Anxiety and fear	Perform common treatment for chest injuries, above. *Specifics:* ☐ Rib fractures are not wrapped, strapped or taped.
Flail chest (when several ribs in the same area are broken in more than one place) ☐ Breathing: painful, the victim may be trying to support the injured area	Perform common treatment for chest injuries, above. *Specifics:* ☐ If the victim is experiencing pain and difficulty breathing: expose and examine the injury, provide support with your hand to the injured area and provide assisted breathing if necessary.
Abdominal injury – Internal bleeding – Illness ☐ LOC: decreased level of consciousness ☐ Breathing: difficult, short of breath ☐ Skin: sweating ☐ Rigidity of abdominal muscles ☐ Nausea and vomiting ☐ Pain in the abdomen ☐ Shock ☐ Anxiety	Perform common treatment for chest injuries, above.
Abdominal injury with protruding organs ☐ Internal organs are visible outside the body, sticking out through the wound	Perform common treatment for chest injuries, above. *Specifics:* ☐ Keep the protrusion from drying – cover the protrusion with a sterile dressing that has been moistened with very clean, preferably sterile water – don't use materials like paper towel, toilet tissue or cotton, which cling when wet. ☐ Protect it from further damage. ☐ Do not try to put the organs back in the abdomen. ☐ Do not give the victim anything to drink or eat.

INTERNAL ILLNESS

Signs and symptoms are not always caused by external forces. In the same way our heart can have a sudden "attack," our internal organs can be sick from underlying medical disorders and cause sudden pain or other symptoms. Consult a doctor if there are symptoms of internal injury.

PNEUMOTHORAX

A pneumothorax is the result of an injury where air gets into the chest cavity. In most cases there is an open wound, but it can also occur as a result of a closed wound such as broken ribs or another internal injury. Pneumothorax may cause one or both lungs to collapse and lead to a life-threatening breathing emergency. If breathing becomes more difficult, a tension pneumothorax may be developing. Tension pneumothorax is a buildup of air that collapses the lung and puts pressure on the heart, which then can't pump blood effectively, and may lead to a serious medical condition. To treat this injury, follow treatment for a sucking chest wound. In the case of a tension pneumothorax, unseal the wound and adjust the dressing, ensuring one end is open.

REPETITIVE STRAIN INJURY (RSI)

Repetitive strain injuries develop over time – perhaps days, weeks, or months – as a result of muscle and tendon overuse. When someone repeats a particular movement again and again, especially a movement that causes stress on the tissues, he or she may develop RSI. Common examples are "tennis elbow" and "carpal tunnel syndrome."

Treatment for RSI is straightforward: stop the activity causing the injury, follow the steps in "RICE," and see a doctor.

Bone and joint injuries

Together, bones and joints create the mechanism for body movement. Bones serve as rigid levers for tendons and muscles. Joints are formed where two or more bones come together and allow flexibility. Freely moving joints are covered with smooth cartilage to minimize friction and are held together by bands of strong tissue called ligaments.

Sprains and strains

Both injuries refer to stretching or tearing the tissues associated with bones and muscles. A sprain is an injury to an overstretched ligament, which holds bones together at a joint, whereas a strain involves overstretching a muscle or tendon.

Treatment is the same whether the area has been sprained or strained, or both. A fracture that does not actually shift the bone out of alignment may mimic a sprain or strain, and only an X-ray can tell for sure, so treat the symptoms.

Common causes of muscle strain include:
- Not warming up before physical activity.
- Poor body mechanics during exercise or while lifting.
- Sudden movements.
- Repetitive, long-term overuse.

Sprains and strains

Signs and symptoms	Treatment
Pain, could be mild or severe Swelling Discolouration (bruising) Difficulty moving the affected area	"RICE" **Rest** – Rest the injured part. **Immobilize** – Immobilize it in a comfortable position – do NOT move it. **Cold** – Ice the injured part for 10–15 minutes every hour until the swelling subsides. Icing is the most important component of treatment. Avoid placing ice directly against skin; wrap it in a cloth. **Elevate** – Elevate an immobilized limb only if it does not increase pain or discomfort. Advise victim to see a doctor for medical follow-up.

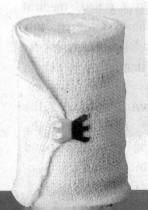

Dislocations and fractures

Some of the twists, hits and falls that cause strains or sprains, can be forceful enough to cause the bones to move out of place or to break. Here are some classifications:

- **Dislocation** – the bones do not break, but they do "pop out" of alignment at the joints. The most common spots are shoulders, fingers and toes.
- **Closed (simple) fractures** – bones break and may shift out of alignment.
- **Open (compound) fractures** – as above, but the bone breaks through the skin.
- **Pelvic/hip fractures** – although not a separate classification because of their location on the body, specific first aid procedures are suggested below.

Dislocations and fractures

Signs and symptoms

Dislocation
- Pain
- Swelling
- Discolouration
- Difficulty moving the affected area
- The joint may look deformed or out of its normal position

Closed fracture
- Pain
- Swelling
- Discolouration
- Difficulty moving the affected area
- Deformity
- Victim may report having heard a cracking sound when incident happened

Femur fracture
- Pain may be severe
- Foot and leg roll outward
- Limb may look deformed and appear shorter than the uninjured limb
- Possible internal bleeding causing severe shock

Open fracture
- Pain
- Swelling
- Discolouration
- Difficulty moving the affected part
- Bone protruding through the skin
- Bleeding wound

Pelvic (hip) bone injuries
- Injury usually involves a large force, perhaps from a fall or motor vehicle crash
- Pain in hips, groin and small of the back
- Pain from pressure to sides of hips
- Cannot lift legs when lying on back
- Deformity
- Urge to urinate (the bladder is the organ most often damaged with a pelvic injury)

Treatment

- Rest the injured part.
- Immobilize it in a comfortable position – do NOT move it.
- Ice the injured part for 10–15 minutes every hour.
- Support the injured part in a comfortable position. Do not attempt to put the bones back; this can cause more damage.
- Phone EMS.

"RICE"
- **Rest** – Rest the injured part.
- **Immobilize** – Immobilize it in a comfortable position – do NOT move it.
- **Cold** – Ice the injured part for 10–15 minutes every hour until the swelling subsides. Icing is the most important component of treatment. Avoid placing ice directly against skin; wrap it in a cloth.
- **Elevate** – Elevate an immobilized limb only if it does not increase pain or discomfort.
- To help breathing, try placing the victim in a semi-sitting position, leaning slightly towards the injured side.
- Phone EMS.
- Assess sensation and circulation above and below the injury. For instance, assess the pulse in the foot if the leg is broken

- Unless it is absolutely essential, do NOT move victims with this condition – it could cause further muscle and nerve damage.
- Rest the affected part.
- Immobilize it as you found it. Do not attempt realignment.
- Place a clean bandage over the exposed bone and wound.
- Note: do not elevate a limb with a fracture.
- Phone EMS.
- Assess sensation and circulation above and below the injury.

- Phone EMS.
- Immobilize in position found.
- Hold hips and support.
- Try not to move or lift legs.
- If in the water, immobilize on a spineboard for removal. (See p. 54)
- Check distal circulation and sensation in the legs.
- Consider possibility of severe internal bleeding, which means call EMS and treat for shock.

Immobilization – dislocation and fractures

Preventing an injured part of the body from moving reduces the chance of further damage and helps minimize pain. Immobilization also includes supporting the injury. Be gentle to avoid a ripple effect of movement from one part to another. If the injury is an "open" fracture, attend to the wound before immobilizing it.

Here are four options for immobilization:

1. Ask the victim to hold the injured part (e.g. arm fracture) carefully against his or her body.

2. Use an arm sling (e.g. hands, wrists, arms, elbows or shoulders). (See page 51).

3. Gently tie the injured part to the body using the body as a splint. Wrap two or three bandages, tying away from the injured site.

   For comfort:
   - Use as wide a bandage as you can find.
   - Pad hollow spaces. Use folded cloth (scarves, kerchiefs, dish towels, etc.) to pad between the limb and the body, especially at the elbow or between legs. Open space leaves room for undesired movement during transport and invites unintentional tightening, which could move the injured part.

   Where to tie:
   - Arms (wrists, hands): tie the bandage around the arm and the torso.
     - Legs (knees, ankles, feet): tie legs together.

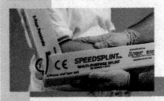
Closed fracture of the forearm.

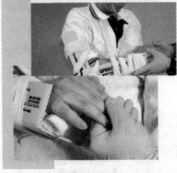

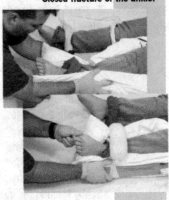
Closed fracture of the ankle.

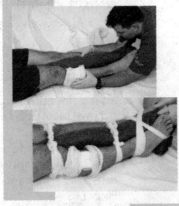
Open fracture of the lower leg.

Closed fracture of the knee.

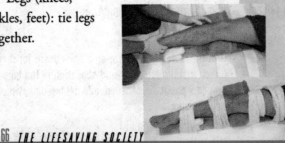

4. Splint: If emergency medical personnel will be transporting the victim, let them handle the splinting. If it is up to the first aiders, here are the basics:

Materials: A variety of objects can serve as a splint, as long as it provides support and keeps injured parts from moving. Consider using items at-hand such as rolled up newspapers, magazines, cardboard, a hockey stick or purchasable air or wooden splints. Pillows and towels work especially well around wrists, ankles and feet. Using other body parts as splints is also effective, such as the finger beside a broken finger.

How to splint:
- Check distal circulation.
- Try to splint the injury in the position found.
- Choose a splint that is long enough. Place it underneath or alongside the fractured area.
- Splint the joints above and below the injury to immobilize. Don't just splint against the injury.
- Secure the splint firmly in place using strips of cloth or bandages tied above and below the injury. The splint should be tied securely enough to prevent movement and provide support.
- Pad the splint so it fits the shape of the body as well as any natural hollows such as behind the knees or in the small of the back. This provides support and comfort.

Afterwards: Check circulation beyond the injury – at the ankle, toes, wrist or fingers. Pinch the finger/toenail: does it return to normal colour when you let go? Is the extremity cold? If colour does not return, or the extremity is cold, you may need to loosen the bandages. Check how the injured limb responds to touch. Numbness or loss of feeling in fingers or toes may indicate nerve damage. Compare it with the uninjured limb.

Burns

Burns are tissue injuries caused by excess heat and cold, or by chemicals, electricity or radiation. Burns can affect more than just body tissue; severe burns can affect all major body systems. Seek medical assistance to properly assess burn damage and watch for these complications:

- shock
- infection
- breathing problems
- swelling

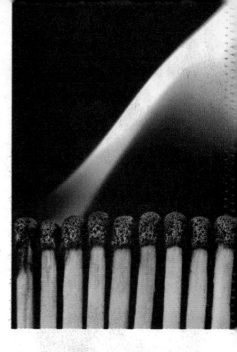

The severity of a burn is determined by:

- the depth (or degree) of the burn
- the amount of burned body surface
- which part(s) of the body is burned
- the age and condition of the victim

Critical burns require immediate medical attention. Seek assistance for:

- burns that interfere with breathing (e.g. throat or face burns, inhalation injuries)
- burns where there is also serious soft tissue injury or a fracture
- all electrical burns
- most chemical burns
- burns to very young or old victims

Most burns can be prevented, so use precautions: keep hot liquids out of reach from children, teach children about heat and electricity dangers, wear eye protection, store chemicals in locked cupboards, and wear protective clothing and sunscreen while in the sun.

Heat ("thermal") burns

Common heat burns are caused by sudden exposure to sources of intense heat such as a flame, gas explosion, or scalding water. There are two categories of heat burns, classified by thickness:

1. Partial thickness burns (affecting the upper layers of skin):
   - First-degree burns affect the surface of the skin. They may cover a small or large area of the body.
   - Second-degree burns affect the upper layers of skin and cause blistering of the skin.
2. Full thickness burns (affecting all layers of the skin):
   - Third-degree burns affect all layers of skin. They may also affect the underlying muscles, nerves and bones.

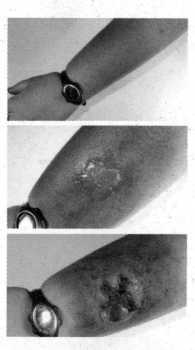

Heat burns

Signs and symptoms	Treatment
First-degree	Flush the burned area with cool, clean water.
Redness	Repeat the flushing until the victim notes that the heat in the affected area has subsided.
Pain	Phone EMS if the area burned is large, the face and neck are affected, or the victim is a small
Mild swelling	child or infant.
Anxiety	
Shock	
Second-degree	Flush the burned area with cool, clean water.
Above, plus:	Cover the affected area with a sterile, dry dressing.
Blisters	Do not break blisters, but if they break on their own, cover with a dry sterile dressing and
	bandage.
	Advise victim to see a doctor for medical follow-up.
	Phone EMS if the area burned is larger than the palm of your hand, the face and neck are
	affected, or the victim is a small child or infant.
Third-degree	Phone EMS.
Above, plus:	Flush the burned area with cool, clean water.
Red, black and grey tissue	Cover the affected area with a sterile, dry dressing.
Waxy tight tissue	Do not break blisters, but if they break on their own, cover with a dry sterile dressing and
Underlying tissue and organs exposed	bandage.
(e.g. muscles, nerves, bones)	If the hands and feet are affected, separate the fingers or toes with dressings.
Pain in severely affected areas may	
be absent if the nerves have been	
damaged	

Chemical burns

There are many chemicals common to either industrial or home settings. Chemical burns can be serious because the substance continues to burn for as long as it remains on the skin. Follow the manufacturer's directions for storing chemicals. Always keep dangerous chemicals in a safe place away from children and keep them in a location where there is minimal danger of accidental spillage.

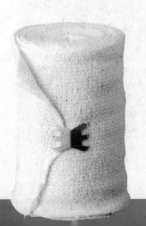

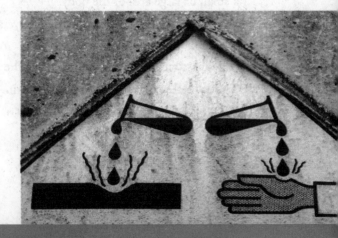

Chemical burns

Hazard prevention: Do not touch chemical products or the container they are in. Wear gloves and use a brush or cloth to avoid coming in contact with the poison. If hazardous material spills, call the fire department.

Signs and symptoms	Treatment
Same as for heat burns	Do not touch chemical products or the container they are in. Wear gloves and use a brush or cloth to avoid coming in contact with the poison.
	Remove contaminated clothing.
	Brush off dry chemicals before flushing with water.
	Flush the area with clean, cool water (not ice-cold water) for at least 15 minutes.
	Use large volumes of water to flush these burns. Start washing the chemical off the skin as soon as possible.
	Phone EMS if the area affected is larger than your palm, the face and neck are affected, or the victim is a small child or infant.
Chemicals in the eye (dry or liquid)	Phone EMS.
	Flush eye with lots of skin-temperature water for at least 30 minutes — flushing should continue during transport to hospital.
	Rinse from the inside to the outside of the eye, including under the lids.
	Encourage the victim to blink constantly while flushing to get under the lid — do NOT lift the eyelid.
	Seek medical attention as soon as possible.

Electrical burns

A spark from any electrical current entering the body can cause injury. Do not underestimate the potential of severe unseen internal damage, even for seemingly small burns.

Electrical burns

Signs and symptoms	Treatment
Distress	Phone EMS.
Breathing and circulation problems: respiratory distress or heart disruption if the shock travels to those areas or to the brain centres controlling those areas	Turn OFF the current before touching the victim or the electrical source. Only EMS or the electrical company should handle high voltage wires and power lines. Do not attempt to use a stick or plastic pole to remove a fallen wire from the victim. Stay well back.
Victim may be without pulse or non-breathing	Stand in a dry area.
Entrance and/or exit wounds (with internal damage in between)	Look for wounds where electricity entered and exited the body, and cover the wounds with a dry dressing.
Burns appear similar to heat burns	
Anxiety, shock	

Radiation burns

Radiant energy emits from sources such as the sun, sunlamps at tanning salons and X-rays.

Sunburn – ranges from mild to severe and can occur on an isolated or large area of the body depending on which areas were left exposed to direct sunlight. Symptoms may develop hours after the exposure.

Intense light burns – caused by direct or reflected sunlight, a welder's flash or snow-blinding. As with sunburn, it may be several hours after the exposure before the victim develops symptoms.

Radiation burns

Signs and symptoms	Treatment
Sunburn	Get out of the sun.
Redness of the affected area	Relieve the affected area with cool water or with a wet towel.
Blistering	Pat dry and apply medicated ointment for sunburns.
	Protect the area from further exposure.
	Do not break blisters.
	If the victim has widespread blistering, seek medical assistance.
	If the victim begins to vomit or develop a fever, treat for heatstroke and seek medical assistance.
Intense light burns	Cover the eyes using a moist cool dressing.
Sensitivity to light	Seek medical assistance.
Pain	
Gritty feeling in the eyes	

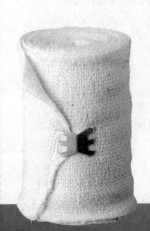

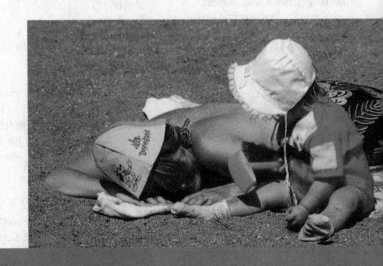

Poisoning

Poisons are substances that can cause illness or death when absorbed by the body. While many poisonous consumer products are labelled as poisons, there are many that do not carry labels such as alcohol, medication taken in improper doses, cleaning products and other common household items. Some of these substances are not harmful in small amounts, but become poisonous in large amounts.

The best way to prevent poisoning is to take precautions. Be sure to:

- read product labels
- throw away food that may be contaminated
- ventilate areas if you use toxic chemicals
- keep drug products in their original containers
- teach your children how to recognize warning labels and other poisonous items like some plants

There are traditionally four types of poisoning:

1. **Ingested**: Eating spoiled or contaminated food, drinking cleaning agents, reaction to medicine, overdose of pills or drugs, eating plants.
2. **Injected**: Injecting prescription or non-prescription drugs, receiving stings from insects.
3. **Inhaled**: Inhaling chemical product powders and vapours, carbon monoxide, car exhaust, chlorine gas and other industrial gases.
4. **Contact (or absorbed)**: Absorbing insecticides, herbicides, plants or pool-water chemicals through the skin.

Poisoning – victim and incident history

If you suspect or know that a poison is involved, ask: "What was taken? When? How much?" Children or adolescents may resist answering. Be persistent. Emphasize the urgent need to fix the situation before it gets worse.

Signs and symptoms	Treatment
LOC: reduced level of consciousness	☐ Phone EMS. ☐ Contact the Poison Information Centre for assistance. (Check the front pages of your telephone book for the local number.)
Ingested ☐ Nausea, abdominal cramps, diarrhea, vomiting ☐ Mouth: discoloured lips, burns around the mouth, breath odour	**Ingested** ☐ Do not induce vomiting unless directed by a doctor or poison control official. ☐ If conscious, wipe poison residue from the victim's face and mouth. ☐ Whenever possible, put the poison and its container in a clear plastic bag. Note the name of the poison, and give that information and the poison container to EMS.
Injected ☐ Irritation at point of entry	**Injected** ☐ Delay circulation by placing the victim at rest and keeping the affected limb below heart level.
Inhaled ☐ Breathing: difficult, coughing ☐ Headache ☐ Changes in behaviour, hallucinations, agitation, drowsiness	**Inhaled** ☐ Remove victim away from the source of any inhaled poisons – do not become a victim. It may be necessary to request and wait for fire department assistance. ☐ Use a face mask or shield to perform rescue breathing. ☐ If the victim vomits, clear out the mouth. ☐ If the victim has convulsions, prevent them from being injured.
Contact (absorbed) ☐ Skin: reddening, sweating, rash, blisters, swelling	**Contact** (absorbed) ☐ Rinse the area with cool water, or brush off any excess if in powder form. ☐ Remove the clothing that had contact with the substance. ☐ Wash the skin thoroughly with soap and water.

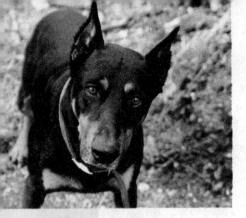

Stings and bites

These injuries are caused by stings or bites from insects, humans or animals. Any bite that breaks the skin is serious and warrants medical attention. Bites from humans and animals are especially dangerous because of the risk of infection.

RABIES

Rabies is an acute viral disease of the nervous system that is fatal if left untreated. You should suspect rabies in domestic animals if they behave unusually (often fearless and aggressive), and in all attacks by wild animals. The virus can be transmitted to anyone who handles a diseased animal or who touches a rabies-contaminated wound. Always wear gloves and wash your hands thoroughly after contact to reduce the risk of infection. Full-blown rabies can be prevented if immunization is given quickly.

Stings and bites – victim and incident history
Does the victim have a history of being allergic to stings? If yes, ask if the victim carries a sting kit (EpiPen®).
If no, this could be the victim's first allergic reaction, so watch for symptoms of anaphylaxis.
What type of animal bit the victim? Does the animal show signs of rabies?

Signs and symptoms	Treatment
General	
Localized pain	**Phone EMS.**
Bleeding	Be certain there is no danger of another attack to the victim
Bruising	or yourself.
Puncture wounds in the skin	
Shock	**Animal or human bites – general**
Breathing: distress, or in some allergic reaction cases, a swelling of the tongue and throat	Examine the wound to determine if the skin is broken. If it is, seek medical assistance as soon as possible.
	If the wound is bleeding moderately, allow it to do so because it is self-cleansing.
	Wash the wound with an antiseptic soap, apply a dressing and bandage.
	Refer to the section on "Wounds" (p. 48–49) for general wound treatment information.
Snakebites	**Snakebites**
Two puncture holes	Immediately apply hand pressure above and below the wound site. Once first aid kit becomes available, apply a pressure bandage to wound and immobilize the limb as for a fracture (see p. 65–66).
Burning sensation	
Swelling, discolouration	
Severe pain	
Weakness, sweating, nausea, vomiting, chills	Place the victim in a semi-sitting position, with the affected limb below heart level – this slows down the spread of venom.
	If possible, flush the bite with soapy water – do not apply ice or a cold compress.
	Seek medical assistance.
Insect bites and stings	**Stings – if no allergic reaction:**
Sudden pain	Monitor breathing.
Swelling	Remove a bee stinger by gently scraping it off skin – do NOT squeeze stinger with tweezers, as this may cause more poison to be injected.
Heat	
Redness, itching	

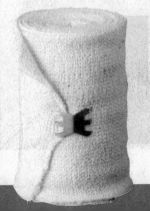

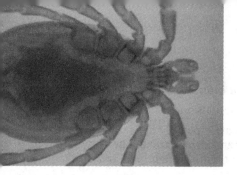

Stings and bites

Signs and symptoms	Treatment
Allergic reaction ■ Itching, rash ■ Bump on the skin – white, pink, red, blotchy ■ Generalized swelling, especially of the airway ■ Weakness, headache ■ Fever ■ Breathing difficulty ■ Anxiety, cramps, vomiting	**Stings – if allergic, or if the victim has difficulty breathing or the air passages swell:** ■ Phone EMS immediately. ■ Help a conscious victim administer an auto-injector – use only the victim's medication, not someone else's. ■ If unconscious, you may administer a victim's own auto-injector. (Use it according to the package instructions. See page 45.) If necessary, the auto-injector will go through clothes. Massage the area to disperse the medication. ■ Try to preserve the insect to assist with identification.
Ticks ■ Tick is embedded in the victim's skin	**Ticks** ■ Use tweezers to grab hold of the tick as close to the victim's skin as possible. If you don't have tweezers use your fingers, but cover them by wearing gloves or use plastic, a tissue, etc. ■ Clean the area with soapy water and apply antiseptic to prevent infection. ■ Seek medical assistance to find out if there is a risk of disease transmission by the ticks in the area. Keep the tick for identification if possible. ■ Seek medical attention if there are any signs of infection.
Leeches ■ Leech is attached to the victim's skin	**Leeches** ■ Do not try to pull the leech off. ■ Detach the leech by applying either salt, heat from a match or lighter, or a drop of kerosene, turpentine or oil to its body – it should fall off on its own. ■ Clean the area with a paste of baking soda and water or a weak solution of ammonia. ■ Seek medical attention if there are any signs of infection.

MARINE LIFE

Marine life injuries are grouped in three main categories:

1. Stings – e.g. jellyfish
2. Punctures – e.g. stingrays
3. Bites – e.g. sharks

For punctures and bites, provide first aid for these types of wounds. For stings, rinse the wound with sea water or, if possible, pour vinegar on it – this helps dissolve stinger cells. Bathe the area in warm water (as warm as the victim can tolerate) for about 20 minutes. Do not apply cold water as this may encourage the stinger cells to continue to release venom. Seek medical assistance.

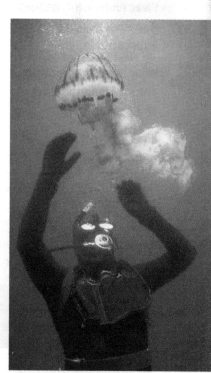

Be Sun-Smart

Overexposure to the sun can be extremely dangerous. In the short term, unprotected exposure can cause moderate to severe sunburn. In the long term, the skin and eyes can be damaged, and the risk of skin cancer and cataracts increases with exposure. Suntans and sunburns are both signs of skin damage. Even after sunburn heals, damage remains and increases with each burn.

Reflections from water, sand, and concrete intensify the effect of the sun's rays. Sunscreen is necessary even on overcast days because the sun's ultraviolet (UV) radiation is still present. Everyone outdoors should take sun-smart precautions:

- Wear protective clothing, and clothing that covers exposed skin.

- Wear a hat that protects the face and the back of the neck.

- Use sunscreen with a sun protection factor (SPF) of at least 30.

- Apply sunscreen and lip balm to protect exposed skin. (Apply and reapply sunscreen according to the manufacturer directions.)

- Wear protective sunglasses.

- Monitor UV ratings and forecasts in weather reports.

Heat cramps

Heat cramps are a result of excess heat and dehydration. The body loses salt and water faster than it can replace them through food and drink.

Heat cramps

Signs and symptoms	Treatment
Abdominal and leg heat cramps	☐ Move to a cool spot out of the hot environment, remove excess clothing.
☐ Victim has been in a hot environment	☐ Give the victim cool water to drink.
☐ Skin: sweating	☐ Stretch the cramp.
☐ Pain and spasms in muscles (particularly in the legs and stomach)	☐ Advise the victim to eat foods that will help restore normal body salt.
☐ Fatigue, dizziness, headache	
☐ Nausea	
☐ Shock	
Muscle cramps from overuse	☐ Stretch the muscle (slowly lengthen the muscle fibres).
☐ Pain in the muscle that has been working or exercising	☐ Gently massage along the length of the muscle.
☐ Muscle twitching or spasms	

Heat exhaustion and heatstroke

Heat exhaustion is another possible reaction to sustained heat and sweating. If left untreated, heat exhaustion can progress into life-threatening heatstroke.

Heatstroke occurs when the body's ability to regulate its temperature fails and the body temperature rises dangerously. Those most likely to suffer heatstroke are young children and infants, the elderly and cardiac patients.

Heat exhaustion and heatstroke

Signs and symptoms	Treatment
Heat exhaustion	☐ Move to a cool spot out of the hot environment.
☐ Hot	☐ Cool the victim gradually (remove as much clothing as possible, bathe with cool water, fan).
☐ Normal mental status – oriented to person, place and time	☐ Cover lightly if victim feels cold.
☐ Nausea, headache, dizziness	☐ If the victim is alert and nausea is not a big problem, give him or her water to drink.
☐ Restlessness, weakness	☐ Advise victim to eat well or consume 'sport' drinks to restore depleted body salt.
☐ Fear, anxiety	☐ Phone EMS if the victim's level of consciousness is decreased.
☐ Confusion, disorientation	
☐ Skin: sweating	
☐ Pulse: weak, rapid	
☐ Respiration: shallow, rapid	
Heatstroke	☐ Phone EMS. This is a life-threatening emergency.
All heat exhaustion signs and symptoms plus:	☐ Move to a cool spot out of the hot environment.
☐ Body temperature rises rapidly	☐ Cool victim down as quickly as possible: cool the body core – head, neck, chest, back, groin – by:
☐ Vomiting, convulsions, unconsciousness	
Classic heatstroke: Skin is flushed, *hot and dry* – body temperature control mechanism fails, sweating stops and body temperature rises quickly	☐ removing outer layer of victim's clothing
	☐ wrapping the victim in wet sheets
	☐ sponging with or immersing in shallow, cool water.
Exertional heatstroke: Skin is flushed, *hot and sweaty* – heavy physical exertion causes body temperature to rise quickly, sweating continues	☐ fanning his or her body
	☐ applying ice packs or cold compresses to head, armpits, groin and along the sides of the chest

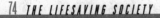

Hypothermia

Hypothermia happens when someone becomes very cold and their core body temperature drops so low that it stops functioning properly.

Often associated with cold weather, hypothermia can also strike when it is relatively warm, especially in damp, windy or rainy conditions. It is also associated with drowning because our bodies lose heat quickly when immersed in cold water. All lakes, streams, rivers and oceans in Canada, during any season, can be considered "cold" – cold enough to trigger hypothermia.

If a mild case of hypothermia is left unattended, the victim's condition can deteriorate to the point where the exposure is severe and life-threatening. The three stages of hypothermia are i) Mild, ii) Moderate, and iii) Severe.

Hypothermia – incident history

Transition from mild to severe symptoms will not necessarily be obvious. Recognize the early signs and act promptly.

Signs and symptoms

Note: This list is in order from mild to severe, but a victim can experience several symptoms at once.

Mild
- Shivering, feeling cold
- Loss of coordination
- Fatigue
- Slurred speech
- Stumbling, loss of muscular coordination
- Shock

Moderate
- Uncontrollable shivering
- Disorientation, confusion, lapses in memory, may appear intoxicated
- Decreased consciousness
- Blurred vision and hallucinations

Severe
- Shivering reduced or absent
- An overwhelming desire to sleep
- Loss of consciousness

Treatment

- Remove victim to a dry, sheltered place.
- Handle gently (avoid jolting or rough handling).
- Do not rub the victim's body surfaces.
- If possible, remove wet clothing and dry victim.
- Warm the victim's body by:
  - giving warm beverages (no alcohol) if the victim is alert
  - wrapping victim in warm blankets
  - getting into the huddle position.
  - applying heat packs to head, neck and trunk
- Phone EMS if the victim is unconscious, confused or does not improve quickly.

PREVENTING HYPOTHERMIA

To prevent the onset of hypothermia, always dress appropriately for the weather and the activity you are doing. Stay safe by using the "buddy system" to check on one another. Stay dry, eat high energy foods (e.g. nuts, dried fruit) and drink plenty of non-caffeinated, alcohol-free liquids. And keep your body moving to create heat.

FROZEN STATE

If the temperature is below zero, it is possible for someone to become completely frozen.

Recognize a frozen person if:

- the victim is found unresponsive and in a cold location
- the joints of the jaw and neck are rigid
- the skin and deeper tissues are cold and cannot be depressed
- the body moves as a solid unit

There is no treatment for a frozen victim – get yourself to safety and call EMS.

Frostbite

Frostbite describes frozen parts of the body. It is a progressive injury with two stages:

1. **Superficial frostbite** – symptoms include pain followed by numbness.

2. **Deep frostbite** – a serious medical condition where the victim has no feeling in the area. The area should be re-warmed in water if medical assistance is not readily accessible.

Frostbite generally starts with exposed skin on the tips of the nose, ears, cheeks and fingers. But it can creep into the toes, feet, hands and face as a person remains out in the cold.

Prevention: It is difficult to monitor frostbite on yourself because you can't always feel it or see it. In cold weather, the best approach is to watch your friends and have them watch you for little white spots on the face. Check every 10 or 15 minutes. Also pay attention to how your feet (or other susceptible body parts) are feeling. If you cannot feel a body part, and have been in the cold for a long time, return to a warm place and complete a visual check.

Frostbite

Signs and symptoms	Treatment
White, waxy look to the affected area	Remove the victim from the cold environment, i.e., go indoors.
Pain	Reheat the affected area:
Loss of feeling, numbness	with body heat (e.g. put frostbitten fingers under the armpits, or cup the frostbitten face or ears in the hands)
Altered sensation, such as burning or pins and needles	or, immerse the affected body part in warm (comfortable to touch) water for 20-30 minutes until the body part is red and warm. The ideal water temperature is 37–40° Celsius.
Skin starts out soft and progressively becomes hard to the touch	Do not rub the area that appears frozen, and do not apply snow.
Joints stiffen	Keep the injury warm and ensure it does not become frozen again. Do not apply chemical warmers (e.g. pocket warmers) directly on frostbitten tissue. The high temperatures they produce can cause more harm, potentially burning the injured tissue.
	Apply a loose, dry dressing (don't break the blisters) to protect the injury.
	Advise victim to seek medical assistance.

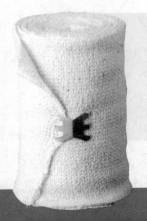

Pressure-related water injuries

Changes in air pressure under water can cause problems for swimmers, skin divers and scuba divers. These pressure changes occur because air compresses below the surface.

Squeezes

A squeeze is similar to ears popping in an airplane during an ascent or descent. Under water, this can affect air cavities in the body besides the ears, such as sinuses, lungs, intestines, and air spaces in dental fillings. "Mask squeeze" occurs while using snorkeling equipment. While squeezes can be quite painful, and some (mask, sinus, ear) may discharge blood, squeezes will usually get better on their own.

Bubble injuries

Lung expansion, bubble injuries, embolisms, decompression sickness and the bends are all life-threatening. Air bubbles may form in a scuba diver's bloodstream while the diver is deep under water. The danger is from those bubbles expanding as the scuba diver returns to the surface.

Pressure-related injuries — incident history

If the victim breathed compressed air under water using scuba equipment, or simply breathed air from a submerged container, then consider the possibility that the compressed air may have caused an injury.

Signs and symptoms	Treatment
Squeezes - Severe pressure pain in the area where the air is trapped - A mask squeeze may leave the eyes bloodshot and a distinctive outline of the mask imprinted on the victim's face	- Monitor victim to make certain they are improving. - Direct victim to consult their doctor. - Phone EMS if the victim is distressed or the condition does not improve.
Bubble injuries - LOC: changes, confusion, disorientation, unconsciousness - Breathing: shortness of breath or coughing - Skin: itch, rash - Localized pain - Joint pain - Weakness, fatigue, dizziness - Paralysis, loss of feeling, blurred vision - Chest pain - Convulsions	- Place victim in recovery position. - Phone EMS and advise them the injury is pressure-related. Provide detailed information from your assessment. If a scuba diver's diving log is available, send it with the victim.

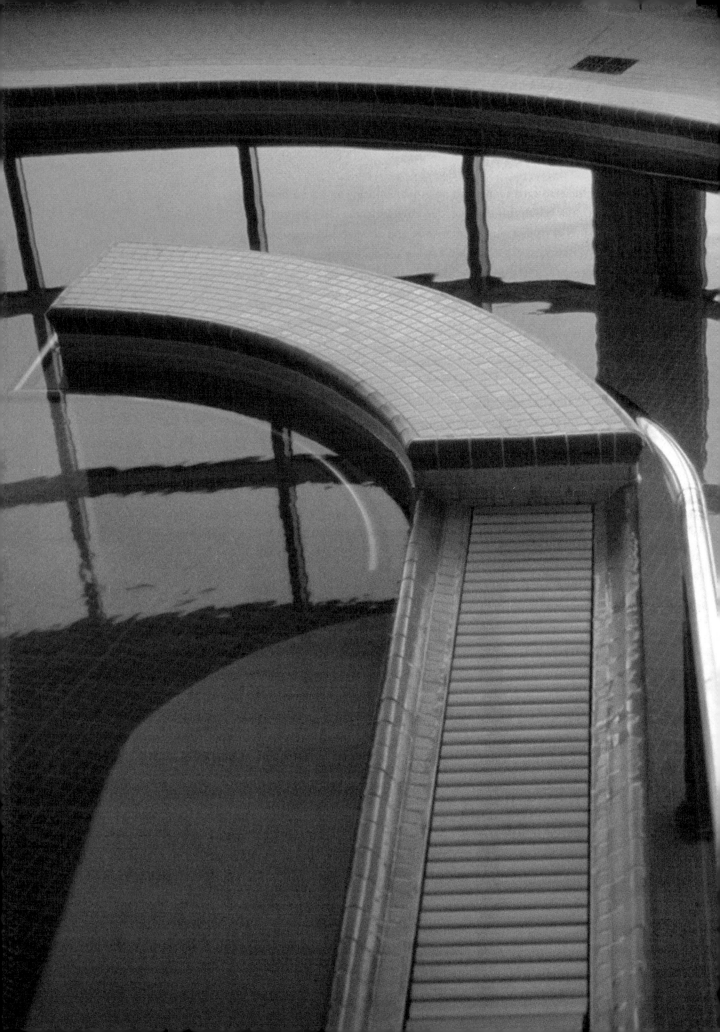

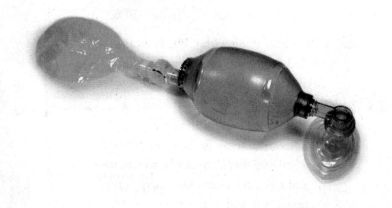

AED AND AIRWAY MANAGEMENT

Canadian Chain of Survival

The survival of a victim of circulatory disease depends upon a series of interventions in the "Canadian Chain of Survival" (see p. 9) When a first aider recognizes cardiac arrest and performs CPR, the first links of the chain are activated. Access to early defibrillation is the next link. The sooner defibrillation occurs, the better a victim's chance of survival.

AED — Protocols

The 2005 revisions to resuscitation guidelines changed the AED protocol. The new AED protocol alternates single shocks with CPR.

A victim who requires defibrillation benefits most from a combination of shocks and chest compressions. When the AED administers a shock, the heart is momentarily stunned and may take several minutes to beat effectively enough to circulate the blood on its own. Performing CPR immediately after a shock helps to circulate the blood while the heart recovers.

Manufacturers are continuously improving their AED units. Follow the prompts provided by the AED unit you are using.

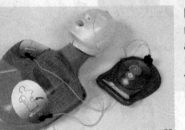

Pad placement on an ACTAR D-fib training manikin.

EQUIPMENT-RELATED TREATMENT

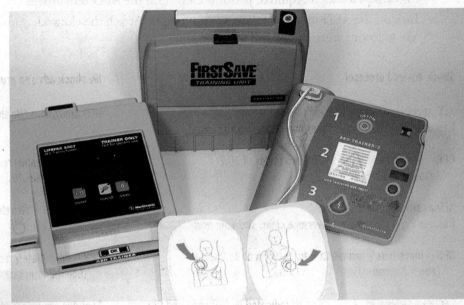

Automated External Defibrillator (AED)

An AED is a sophisticated computerized device designed to restore the normal rhythm of the heart with an electric shock. AEDs are now accessible to the public through the development and use of portable AEDs.

Using the AED, along with CPR, is recommended for victims of cardiac arrest. Survival rates are significantly higher when both CPR and AED are administered.

- **"Automated"** means the unit monitors electrical activity in the heart, advises whether a shock should be administered, and sets a corresponding energy dose that is safe and effective.

- **"External"** means it is attached to the chest, not directly to the heart.

- Fibrillation is a quivery, vibratory movement of the heart muscle, which is usually fatal – **"Defibrillation"** reverses that quivering.

The first aider only has to know:

- when to use the AED unit
- basic steps to operate the AED unit

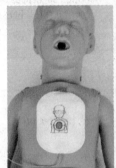

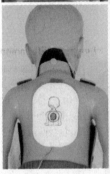

If the child is small, place pads so as not to touch each other. Place one on the front and one on the back.

AED – Protocols

- Assess the scene and victim responsiveness. If victim is unresponsive, call EMS and send for the AED unit.
- Check ABCs and, if required, perform CPR until the AED unit arrives.
- Turn on the AED unit and follow voice prompts. Attach the electrode pads to the victim's bare chest. One of the following instructions will apply.

Shock advised protocol	No shock advised protocol
AED analyzes – "Shock advised" Rescuer says: "Stand clear; everyone clear; shocking now."	AED analyzes – "No shock advised"
CPR – Immediately resume CPR for 5 cycles of 30:2 (about 2 minutes).	CPR – Immediately resume CPR for 5 cycles of 30:2 (about 2 minutes).
AED analyzes – "Shock advised" Rescuer says: "Stand clear; everyone clear; shocking now."	AED analyzes – "No shock advised"
CPR – Immediately resume CPR for 5 cycles of 30:2 (about 2 minutes).	CPR – Immediately resume CPR for 5 cycles of 30:2 (about 2 minutes).
Continue sequences of one shock (if indicated by AED unit) and CPR until medical help arrives or given other AED prompts. If "no shock advised" is indicated, go to **No shock advised protocol.**	Continue sequences of CPR and analyzing until victim recovers or medical help arrives or given other AED prompts. If shock is advised at any time go to **Shock advised protocol.**

Automated External Defibrillator (AED) – How to operate

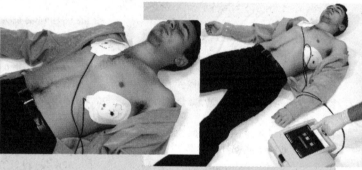

Signs and symptoms

- LOC: unresponsive
- Breathing: non-breathing

Treatment

- Phone EMS.
- Get the AED unit.
- Remove clothing covering chest.

Common AED components

- On/Off button (some units automatically turn on if opened)
- Analyze button (most units will automatically check for a "shock-able" rhythm once attached)
- Shock button (delivers a shock to the victim if pushed)
- Defibrillation pads and cables (many come with diagrams instructing you where to place them on the victim)
- Batteries
- Audible alarms and prompts
- Visual alarms and prompts

Operating steps

- Turn the power* switch "on" or lift up the monitor cover. The AED will prompt you through the steps using voice prompts, or a screen that displays messages.
- Position electrodes on victim and connect to AED (look for a diagram on the AED). The pads are self-adhesive. If the AED prompts indicate "check electrodes," ensure the pads are firmly attached to the chest and the cables are secured to the AED unit. Make sure the victim is dry and if there is hair on the chest, shave it.
- Respond to voice prompts and machine indicators.
- Analyze the rhythm – no one should touch the victim – movement may cause an inaccurate analysis. If the AED prompts indicate "motion detected," have everyone stay still and be sure no one is touching the victim. The most common cause is the rescuer moving near the victim or the victim is breathing.
- Follow the AED protocol for **shock advised** or **no shock advised** as indicated by the unit:
  - **Shock advised:** call "clear!" and do a visual check to ensure no one is in contact with the victim. Push the shock button. Expect to see sudden muscular contraction of the chest. Immediately resume CPR starting with chest compressions. Do 5 cycles of 30:2 (about 2 minutes). Re-analyze and follow AED instructions.
  - **No shock advised:** immediately resume CPR starting with chest compressions. Do 5 cycles of 30:2 (about 2 minutes). Re-analyze and follow AED instructions.
- Transfer care to EMS personnel. Provide written and verbal reports.

* If the AED prompts indicate "low battery," the unit only has limited power. Follow the manufacturer's directions.

AED – Other considerations

If this present...	then modify AED by:
Water, in pools or if victim is wet	Remember, water conducts electricity. Excessive moisture on the skin can decrease the effectiveness of the shock. Be sure to: • Remove victim from freestanding water and move to a dry area. • Ensure the victim's chest is dry, and that you are dry.
Victim is under 8 years of age or under 25 kg (55 lbs.)	When assisting children less than 8 years of age, focus on supporting airway and breathing, since most causes of arrest in children are related to trauma or breathing problems versus sudden cardiac arrest. Some AEDs are equipped to handle child victims – typically they use a different set of child pads and may adhere to the front and back of the victim – check with your equipment manual and the supplier. If you are giving CPR to a child (1 to 8 years) and the available AED does not have child pads or a way to deliver a smaller dose, use a regular AED with adult pads. DO NOT use child pads or a child dose for adult victims in cardiac arrest. Continue CPR.
Medicine patches on chest	Chest medical patches, such as nitroglycerine patches for angina patients, should be removed if they are in the way of applying AED pads and the area wiped clean. If the patch is not removed, it may block the energy delivered through the pads and cause burning. Wear gloves and handle the patch carefully to avoid contact with the medication. Attach electrodes once the area is clean.
Hairy chest	If the victim has excessive chest hair (i.e., the pads do not stick to the skin), shave the area where the pads will be placed to ensure they adhere properly.
Implanted pacemakers • hard lump beneath the skin of upper chest or abdomen (usually on the left side) • the size of a half-deck of cards • may be a small scar	Place the electrode pad at least 2.5 cm (1 in.) away. *Automated Implantable Cardio Defibrillators (AICD)* Some people have a small device implanted in their torso that delivers automatic shocks to the heart. Attach the AED pads in the same manner as for pacemakers, making sure they are 2.5 cm (1 in.) away. If you see minor contractions in the area while you are readying the AED, wait 20–30 seconds until the AICD is finished. You can touch the victim while the AICD is shocking.
Oxygen rich environments	Remove oxygen from the victim when administering a shock.
Electrocution	Continue with the same AED protocols if the victim was struck by lightning or suffered from another form of electrocution.
Vomit	If the victim vomits at the same time the AED indicates a shock, continue with AED protocol, administering a shock followed by clearing the airway of vomit or fluids.
Pregnancy	The best way to save the baby is to save the mother. Continue AED protocols.

If two rescuers...	then:

Rescuer 1	**Rescuer 2**
• phones EMS and fetches AED unit (or recruits a bystander). • returns and operates the AED.	• performs primary assessment and begins CPR. • performs CPR.

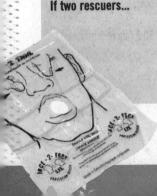

More about AEDs

- Several models of AEDs are available. Should you have occasion to purchase an AED, talk to local EMS personnel – they should be able to give you practical consumer advice.

- If your worksite (or recreation area) has an AED, become familiar with it by reading the directions. Label it clearly and distinctly, know where it is kept and be able to explain its whereabouts to a bystander. Add regular AED review to your in-services and consult with your training agency for the recommended level and frequency of retraining required.

- Ask EMS personnel to help you develop reporting procedures for the emergency site. Expect to report on the number of shocks given, medications used, what happened, and the condition of the victim preceding the incident. When EMS takes over from you at an emergency scene, you want the transition to be as smooth as possible.

- Perform routine checks. As with any first aid equipment, establish a routine to ensure the unit is working well. Follow manufacturer's directions for maintenance. At the least, inspect the AED electrode pads, cables, case, batteries and accessories routinely. Ensure expiration dates for pads and batteries have not passed. Keep it clean and organized.

- **Use of AED on infants:** The need for defibrillation on infants is uncommon, and the preferred treatment involves the use of a manual defibrillator by trained health care professionals. In an emergency, an AED could be used on an infant. If so, use pediatric pads if available. Otherwise, use adult pads.

Location:

- *Personal use:* Family, friends and roommates may consider having an AED for people at high risk of sudden cardiac arrest.

- *Public access:* An increasing number of communities are distributing AEDs in airports, shopping malls, office or housing complexes, golf courses, recreation and fitness centres, and seniors centres.

HEART RHYTHMS AND AED

Normal Sinus Rhythm: Electrical activity of the heart muscle is coordinated, resulting in normal muscle contractions that produce a pulse.

Ventricular Fibrillation (VF): Electrical activity of the heart muscle is uncoordinated, resulting in uncoordinated quivering muscle contractions with no detectable pulse. The AED unit will indicate a shock is advised.

Pulseless Ventricular Tachycardia (VT): Electrical activity of the heart muscle is very rapid and uncoordinated. Atriums and ventricles of the heart muscle do not completely fill with blood, resulting in no detectable pulse. The AED unit will indicate a shock is advised.

Pulseless Electrical Activity (PEA): Electrical activity of the heart muscle is coordinated but the heart muscle is unable to contract or produce a pulse due to some form of severe trauma, such as massive blood loss. The AED unit will not indicate a shock is advised.

Asystole (Flat line): There is no electrical activity of the heart muscle and no muscle contractions producing a pulse. The AED unit will not indicate a shock is advised.

OXYGEN ADMINISTRATION

Introduction

Oxygen administration is about supplying oxygen gas (not just regular air) to a victim. A first aider hooks a tank of oxygen to a face mask with an oxygen inlet, and the victim breathes through that face mask. Oxygen can be used for both breathing and non-breathing victims.

Providing oxygen to a victim is useful to promote recovery. If either breathing or blood circulation is impaired, oxygen is not reaching the body's cells fast enough or in sufficient amounts. By enriching the amount of oxygen in each breath, more reaches the cells where it is needed. Victims who receive oxygen may find it easier to breathe;

it can reduce pain, return skin to a normal colour, reduce a rapid pulse rate and improve the level of consciousness.

You can use oxygen to supplement treatment for a drowning victim, decompression sickness, carbon monoxide poisoning, respiratory arrest, or for victims who warrant the administration of oxygen indicated by a pulse oximeter. A victim with a pulse oximetry reading of less than 94% oxygen should receive oxygen. (See page 88, Pulse Oximetry).

Hypoxia

Hypoxia is a deficiency of oxygen in the body. Anoxia is a complete lack of oxygen.

Hypoxia

Signs and symptoms	Treatment
LOC: confusion, disorientation, unconsciousness **Breathing:** shortness of breath, rapid or ineffective breathing **Circulation:** rapid pulse Anxiety Nausea and vomiting Weakness Shock Seizures	1) Clear the area of explosive hazards like cigarettes, open flames, oil and petroleum products. 2) Assemble the pocket mask: insert the one-way valve and attach the oxygen tubing to the mask. 3) Turn the oxygen tank on and adjust the oxygen flow rate to 10–15 l/minute. Continually monitor the victim's breathing and other vital signs. The use of oxygen should never delay resuscitation including opening the airway, rescue breathing, or chest compressions.
Not breathing	**Steps 1–3 from above, then:** 4) Kneel near the top of the victim's head and place the pocket mask over the victim's face. Start by placing the rim of the mask between the chin and mouth, then lower it to cover the nose and mouth. 5) Seal the pocket mask by placing your thumbs on each side of the mask. Keep the airway open by tilting the head back and placing fingers from both hands along the victim's jawbone. 6) Begin rescue breathing: blow through the mouth piece on the mask.

While administering oxygen to a breathing victim

If...	Then:
1) The rate of breathing decreases 2) Breathing stops altogether 3) Victim vomits	1) Be prepared to assist with rescue breathing. 2) Perform rescue breathing. 3) Remove the mask, clear the airway. Remove foreign matter from the mask by shaking it. Resume administering oxygen.

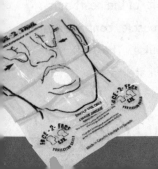

About oxygen equipment

Mask: Use the face mask that comes with the oxygen kit or the same pocket mask you might use as a barrier device. The pocket mask has three openings for air:

1. The mouthpiece where the rescuer puts his or her mouth.
2. Vent holes where the air escapes as the victim exhales.
3. An oxygen adapter port that is similar to an inflation valve on an air mattress. Remove the cover and attach the tubing from the oxygen tank.

Care and safety

Disease transmission: Follow the directions that come with the masks. Do not reuse – most masks are to be discarded after use. Use gloves.

Oxygen tank: The oxygen tank (or cylinder) is similar to a scuba tank, except it is smaller and is filled with pressurized oxygen 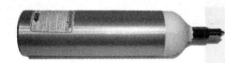 instead of pressurized air. There are two common cylinder sizes for first aiders:

1. D – contains 350 litres of oxygen
2. E – contains 625 litres of oxygen

Oxygen regulator: This device is used with the oxygen tank to control the flow rate. It has a gauge that indicates the amount of oxygen in the tank. The regulator fits onto the oxygen tank "medical post" – the main valve for opening and closing the tank.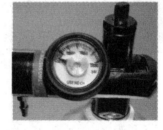

Flow rates: The cylinder operates with simple free flow oxygen. The tank releases a steady flow of air that the victim breathes in as necessary. Any extra flow will escape out the vents of the mask. The rescuer adjusts the rate of flow depending on the needs of the victim and oxygen device. There is no difference for adults, children or infants (assuming the mask fits).

Caution – oxygen tanks contain compressed gas – the pressure inside equals 2000 or 2200 pounds per square inch (PSI).

1. Read and follow the instructions and safety precautions.
2. Only use in conjunction with a regulator.
3. Have the cylinder inspected regularly (and repaired if necessary) by professionals, according to the instructions.
4. Never drop or roll containers. Place them on their side when not in use.
5. Never stand oxygen cylinders on their ends unless they are firmly attached to a wall or other secure structure.
6. Always store them with the valve turned off, with no pressure in the regulator, and in a cool, ventilated dry room.
7. Establish a routine to check and test the unit. Keep regulators and containers clean and in good condition.
8. Even the smallest spark can ignite in an oxygen rich environment. Avoid heat, fire and smoking around oxygen equipment.
9. Using oil or other petroleum products on or around an oxygen device is dangerous. Under pressure, this combination can be explosive. Do not oil the unit for maintenance.

Oxygen delivery

Oxygen device	Common flow rate	Delivers oxygen	Type of victim
Nasal cannula	1–4 litres per minute (lpm)	24–36%	Breathing
Simple face mask	10–15 lpm	35–60%	Breathing
Pocket mask	10–15 lpm	35–60%	Breathing or non-breathing
Bag-valve-mask and Reservoir	10–15 lpm	90% +	Breathing or non-breathing

ADVANCED AIRWAY MANAGEMENT

OROPHARYNX

The oropharynx is the lower portion of the pharynx. The pharynx is at the back of the mouth. It leads into the oesophagus (food pipe) and larynx (voice box), and also communicates with the nose and ears through various tubes.

Oropharyngeal airways

An oropharyngeal airway is a device used to assist in maintaining an open airway. It is a "C-shaped" plastic tube designed to fit inside the throat to prevent the tongue from blocking the airway.

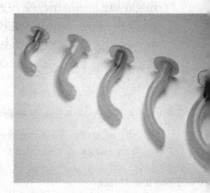

Oropharyngeal airways are not necessary for rescue breathing or oxygen administration and are not recommended for use by most rescuers. Use them only if you have training and have maintained your skill. Opening and maintaining an airway using the head-tilt/chin-lift method works very well.

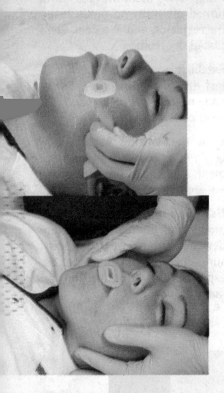

Oropharyngeal airways

Signs and symptoms	Treatment
Unconscious	Check and clear foreign material from the mouth.
	Size the airway – measure the distance from the corner of the victim's mouth to the "angle" of the jaw, where you can feel the corner of jawbone below the ear.
	Open mouth, insert the device upside down.
	When it reaches the end of the mouth, start turning it right-side up as you continue to insert it. Stop when the flange (mouth end) reaches the lips.
	Maintain head position.

If this happens...	then respond...
Adult or child	The tube comes in assorted sizes suitable for anyone.
If victim gags	Remove the oropharyngeal airway immediately.
If victim vomits	Remove the oropharyngeal airway immediately.
	Clear vomit from airway.
	Maintain airway using a regular manual method.
If suspected spinal	Open airway with head-tilt/chin-lift and then insert device.
If victim regains consciousness	Remove it if not tolerated.

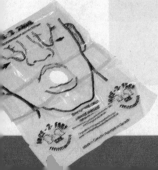

Suction devices

The purpose of a suction device is to clear the airway of fluids and vomit. It is imperative to clear the fluid to keep the airway clear, and to prevent the victim from choking or breathing it back into the lungs. The device acts as a heavy-duty pump for "vacuuming" large chunks of partially digested food, blood clots, blood or any other fluid that pools in a victim's throat. This matter is collected in a bottle incorporated into the design.

Using a suction device is only one method of draining fluids from the mouth. It is not recommended to use one unless you have training and have maintained your skills. The standard method is to place the victim in the recovery position to allow for natural drainage. As you are monitoring vital signs, pay attention to any regurgitation or gurgling. Check for foreign matter in the mouth and clear it out using a hooked finger.

You can use a suction device for unconscious, semi-conscious or conscious victims, but use it with caution in case it triggers vomiting. The advantage of a suction device is it can be less messy and more thorough by reaching to the back of the throat. The suction device needs to have wide-bore tubing, i.e., tubing big enough to accommodate chunks of food without plugging the device.

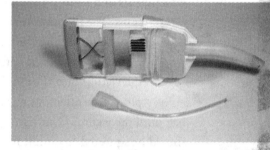

There are a variety of models to choose from. Manual devices powered by pumping with the hands or feet are recommended because of the control you have over the amount of suction.

How to use a suction device

- If you are using it to suction the pharynx, the tip should be contoured to fit over the back of the tongue.
- Place the suction tip before turning on the suction.
- Suction for no more than 15 seconds at a time – suction only what you can see.
- Repeat as necessary, with at least a 15-second interval between suctions.

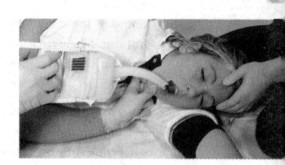

Equipment maintenance

- Read and follow all manufacturer directions.
- Establish a routine to check that the device is in working condition.
- Keep the device clean.

Bag-valve-mask (BVM)

This is a handheld device. Its primary purpose is to ventilate victims who are non-breathing, but it may also be used for victims who are having trouble breathing.

The device has three main components: i) a bag, ii) a valve, and iii) a mask. The bag is self-inflat-

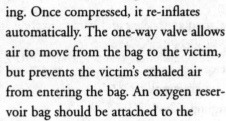

ing. Once compressed, it re-inflates automatically. The one-way valve allows air to move from the bag to the victim, but prevents the victim's exhaled air from entering the bag. An oxygen reservoir bag should be attached to the BVM when supplemental oxygen is administered.

Two-rescuer BVM is preferred, since one rescuer is then free to use two hands to hold the mask, while the second rescuer focuses on ventila-

tions. The first rescuer positions the mask, opens the victim's airway, and maintains a tight seal with the mask on the victim's face. The second rescuer provides ventilations by squeezing the bag until the victim's chest rises. The bag should be squeezed smoothly, not forcefully.

Rescuers responding alone should use mouth-to-

mask technique. CPR with bag-mask ventilation is most effective when performed by two trained and experienced providers. Single-rescuer BVM technique may be used if there is an additional rescuer available to support CPR.

When one rescuer uses the BVM, create a "C-clamp" with your index finger and thumb and place it around the mask. Maintain an open airway using your other finger to lift the jaw. You can use your knees to help hold the victim's head in this tilted position. With one hand, press down on the mask to maintain a tight seal. With your other hand, squeeze the bag slowly until the victim's chest rises.

Nasal cannula

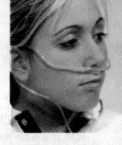

This apparatus delivers oxygen through the victim's nostrils. It is a plastic tube with two small prongs that are inserted into the nose. The use of a nasal cannula is limited, since it is normally used at a relatively low flow rate of 1–4 lpm. This device is not appropriate for a victim experiencing serious respiratory distress, or if the victim's sinuses are blocked by an injury, obstruction or common cold.

Non-rebreathing mask

This equipment delivers oxygen through a mask covering the victim's mouth and nose. The

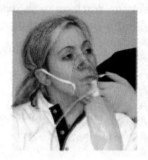

mask contains a reservoir bag and is connected to an oxygen source at a flow rate of at least 10 lpm. A non-rebreathing mask is used on breathing victims only.

Pulse oximetry

A pulse oximeter measures how much oxygen the blood is carrying (SpO_2), shown as a percent age (e.g. 94%). It works by calculating the absorption of red and infrared light in the blood of your fingertip.

- **Using a pulse oximeter:** place on victim's ring or index finger. A percentage of total oxygen saturation is detected and displayed.

- **False readings** may result if there is nail polish, cold hands, significant movement, bright lights affecting the oximeter or if the victim suffers from carbon monoxide poisoning.

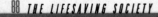

INDEX

NOTES

NOTES

NOTES

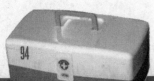

NOTES

NOTES

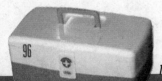

NOTES

NOTES

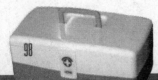